HEART ATTACKS

Are Not Worth Dying For

HEART ATTACKS

Are Not Worth Dying For

Michael Ozner, M.D.

gatekeeper press™

Heart Attacks Are Not Worth Dying For

Library of Congress Control Number: 2020947910

ISBN (paperback): 9781662905353
eISBN: 9781662905360

To my wife Christine
and my children
Jennifer and Jonathan:
You are my heart and soul.

Contents

Foreword

We have made tremendous strides in our treatment of heart and vascular disease over the past decade. Catheter-based techniques are utilized to open occluded coronary arteries, replace heart valves, place stents in aortic aneurysms, and even remove clots from arteries in the brain to treat acute strokes. However, despite the great benefits of interventional techniques, cardiovascular disease remains the leading cause of death for men and women both in the United States and worldwide.

Dr. Michael Ozner, a renowned preventive cardiologist, presents a new approach to prevent cardiovascular disease. This pathway to heart health relies on a healthy lifestyle with optimal nutrition and regular exercise. It also includes maintaining optimal levels of cholesterol and triglycerides to prevent coronary heart disease. Recent clinical research has emerged that now allows physicians to utilize new medications in addition to lifestyle intervention to safely achieve low levels of cholesterol and triglycerides. This novel approach has been shown to stabilize, reverse, and in some cases, eradicate the buildup of fatty deposits in our artery walls called atherosclerotic plaques and thereby lower the risk of heart attack and other vascular catastrophes.

This new book provides the reader with easy-to-understand basics of the underlying problems and importantly presents a clear pathway to heart health. I congratulate Dr. Ozner for introducing a proactive heart disease prevention plan to all interested in achieving optimal health and longevity.

Barry T. Katzen, M.D., FACR, FACC, FSIR
Founder and Chief Medical Executive of
Miami Cardiac & Vascular Institute
Chief Medical Innovation Officer for
Baptist Health South Florida

Introduction

When I first met Suzanne many years ago, she was a seemingly healthy patient. A teacher in her late forties with a teenage daughter, she wasn't the face of heart disease. She was of normal weight and was clearly living an active and productive life. But inside, something was brewing. She had already suffered a mild heart attack and had undergone several stents in her coronary arteries before she came to me seeking help. Her husband had been tragically killed in an automobile accident several years earlier. And now, as a single mother and widow, Suzanne was terrified of "What if . . . ?" What if the treatments and medications didn't work and she had another heart attack? What if she didn't survive? She asked me, "Who will raise my daughter? What can I do?"

If you have ever asked yourself the same questions, yet had no way to answer them, I have news for you. And it is good news. There is much you can do to keep your good health, and even reverse bad health and heart disease. And I am about to tell you how.

For many years I had been intrigued why people living near the Mediterranean Sea, by all accounts, were living healthier lives than Americans. Despite a less advanced medical system, significantly fewer people were dying from heart attacks, cancer, or suffering from chronic conditions like diabetes or Alzheimer's disease. The evidence as to why pointed almost exclusively to their diet and lifestyle.

Chances are, however, that if you're reading this right now, you are frightened of the question "What if . . .?" The hard truth is you likely have good reason to be.

Heart disease is the number one killer in the United States, regardless of gender. And heart disease kills more people each year than all cancers combined. The majority of all of the readers of this book will die of cardiovascular disease (heart attack or stroke) if they don't reverse course. The amazing thing is that heart disease isn't the inevitable consequence of aging. We know what to do to prevent it. And we now know what to do to reverse it!

Unfortunately, our modern "go, go, go" world has, tragically, become "bad, bad, bad" for our health and wreaked havoc on our bodies. Processed foods meant to be "fast" and "convenient" have turned out to be loaded with saturated fat, trans fat, salt, refined starches, and sugar. They are also devoid of essential nutrients. We have replaced the best foods we can eat (e.g., whole, natural foods that are high in good fats, healthy fiber, and free radical fighting antioxidants) with a highly processed, calorie-dense, and nutrient-deficient diet.

Technological advances, while keeping us connected, have rendered us desk-bound, couch-bound, sedentary, stressed, and forgetful on how positively uplifting movement and flexibility are. The result? More and more of us are facing obesity, diabetes, heart disease, cancer, and the inevitable question of "What if . . .?"

Fortunately, we have learned much over the last two decades. Important, life-saving research has shown you can *prevent and even reverse* heart disease and live without the fear of suffering a heart attack. And best of all, this can be accomplished without surgery or catheter-based intervention.

And remember Suzanne, the frightened single mother of a teenage girl, who had a heart attack and underwent multiple coronary angioplasties? I started her on my prevention plan. She changed her diet, started a walking program, began meditation, and stopped smoking. I significantly lowered her "bad" (LDL) cholesterol with a heart-healthy lifestyle and cholesterol-lowering medications. I normalized the number of bad (atherogenic) particles in her blood. I also lowered her marker of vascular inflammation. Most importantly, I gave her hope. She soon realized that she had control of her destiny, and she became healthier and happier. Twelve years later, when she came to my office for her routine annual follow-up, she was smiling and had tears of joy in her eyes as she showed me pictures of her daughter's wedding.

The sad truth is that Americans don't follow a healthy lifestyle or know their risk factors for heart disease. Cardiovascular disease, which includes heart attack, stroke, and vascular disease, kills more than eight hundred thousand Americans each year and is responsible for annual health care costs of nearly half a trillion dollars. Cardiovascular disease is also the leading cause of death for men and women worldwide. Despite these grim statistics, you will be shocked to learn that this deadly disease is actually preventable. As a preventive cardiologist, I have been in the trenches, fighting this disease for decades. We have recently made tremendous progress in our ability to identify and remove the root cause of this disease and the risk factors that flame the fires of this epidemic. My approach is not based on hope or hype but rather well-conducted clinical trials that have paved the way for the scientific community to finally prevent and reverse this mortal enemy. Each chapter will outline the critical information you need to know so you can discuss a heart disease prevention strategy with your personal treating physician. Being proactive against cardiovascular disease will allow you to live a long and heart-healthy life.

CHAPTER 1

A New Approach to Eradicate Heart Disease

Albert Einstein once said, "Insanity is doing the same thing over and over again and expecting a different result."

Despite the billions of dollars being spent on heart disease prevention and intervention, it is still the number one killer of Americans. What we are doing in medicine is not working, and there needs to be a paradigm shift in the way we prevent heart disease. It is often said that people would be able to prevent this devastating disease if they would only follow a healthy lifestyle. Sadly, the reality is that most people are not compliant with healthy lifestyle choices, and sometimes lifestyle changes are not enough to stop the devastation of heart disease.

The good news is that there has been a "revolution" in heart disease prevention over the past decade. This has resulted in major breakthroughs in our battle against heart attack risk factors. Indeed, we have turned the corner, as there is now sufficient research to conclude that cardiovascular disease (heart attack, stroke, and vascular disease) can be prevented and does not have to be the leading killer of men and women in the United States and worldwide.

In this book I'm going to provide you with a roadmap on how to prevent heart disease. An overview of the critical information that you will learn in the chapters to follow is summarized below. This information will be invaluable when you discuss a heart disease prevention strategy with your personal treating physician.

Key Points

> Heart disease is the leading cause of death for men and women worldwide.

> What we are doing to halt this disease is not working. A new approach is needed to prevent atherosclerotic heart and vascular disease.

> Reducing residual risk factors will lower the risk of heart attack and stroke. These risk factors include poor lifestyle habits such as a sedentary lifestyle, a highly processed unhealthy diet, obesity, high blood pressure, smoking, mental stress, insulin resistance and diabetes, elevated lipoprotein (a), and vascular inflammation.

> The primary or root cause of this disease is an excessive number of cholesterol and

triglyceride carrying lipoprotein particles in the circulation; they enter the blood vessel wall and eventually lead to an atherosclerotic plaque (a buildup of cholesterol and fats in the artery wall). When these plaques rupture, a heart attack often occurs.

➢ Low-density lipoprotein (LDL) cholesterol levels are a marker of the number of potentially harmful cholesterol carrying lipoproteins.

➢ Lower is better—the lower the LDL cholesterol we can achieve with a healthy diet and medications (when needed), the lower the risk of heart attack and vascular disease.

➢ Earlier is better—the earlier in life we can achieve a lower LDL cholesterol, the better.

➢ Achieve optimal LDL cholesterol (50 mg/dl to 70 mg/dl throughout life or less than 50 mg/dl to regress or shrink existing atherosclerotic plaques).

➢ Triglycerides, like cholesterol, also increase heart attack risk. Normal triglyceride level is less than 150 mg/dl, and optimal triglyceride level is less than 100 mg/dl.

➢ A landmark clinical trial recently demonstrated that lowering elevated triglyceride levels in patients at high cardiovascular disease risk, who also had optimal LDL cholesterol, significantly lowered major adverse cardiovascular events (including heart attacks and strokes).

> Genetics has paved the way for new medications that now allow us to safely achieve low levels of LDL cholesterol, triglycerides, and lipoprotein (a) that heretofore we were unable to achieve.

> We are now at the dawn of a new era in our quest to defeat cardiovascular disease in the United States and worldwide.

Heart disease is not an inevitable consequence of aging - it can be prevented. Let's get started on the path that leads to a heart-healthy life.

CHAPTER 2

The Primary Cause of a Heart Attack

We can prevent coronary heart disease by attacking and eliminating the primary cause—an excess number of cholesterol and triglyceride carrying particles called lipoproteins.

When there are too many lipoprotein particles in the bloodstream, they can enter the blood vessel wall and lead to an atherosclerotic plaque. A heart attack is the result of a plaque rupture. Genetic studies have paved the way for innovative medications that can lower cholesterol and triglycerides to levels that we previously were unable to achieve. This new therapeutic approach has led to a revolution in the stabilization, regression, and, in some cases, complete elimination of the atherosclerotic plaques. This approach has been shown to significantly reduce heart attacks, strokes, and vascular death.

What is an atherosclerotic plaque?

An atherosclerotic plaque is a collection of cholesterol, fats, and inflammatory cells within the artery wall. When the plaque becomes inflamed, it can rupture and lead to a heart attack.

To better understand the role of cholesterol and inflammation in the development of an atherosclerotic plaque, I have included easy-to-understand illustrations of this process.

Cholesterol and triglycerides produced in the liver are released into the circulation in particles called apoB lipoproteins. These lipoproteins are capable of entering the blood vessel wall, leading to atherosclerotic plaque formation.

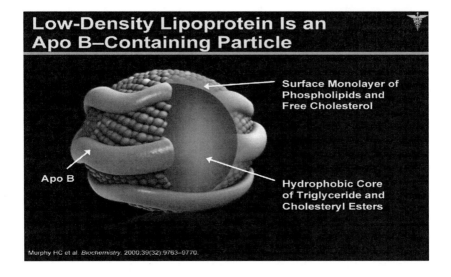

Ninety percent of apoB particles within the bloodstream are LDL (low-density lipoprotein) particles, which carry mainly cholesterol.

LDL particles squeeze through to the lining of the artery wall and become retained and oxidized.

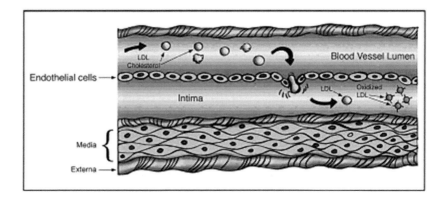

The oxidized cholesterol is then engulfed by inflammatory cells called macrophages.

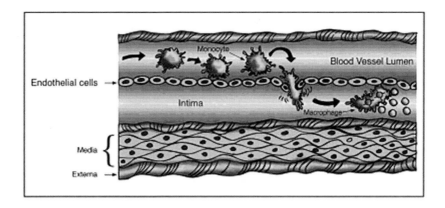

Proteinases (enzymes that breakdown proteins) produced by inflammatory cells break down the fibrous cap of the atherosclerotic plaque, leading to plaque rupture.

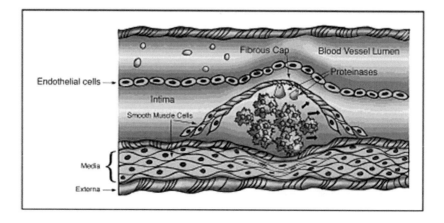

Upon rupture, tissue factor within the plaque, along with platelets, cause blood to clot, blocking flow in the artery. This can lead to a sudden vascular event such as a heart attack.

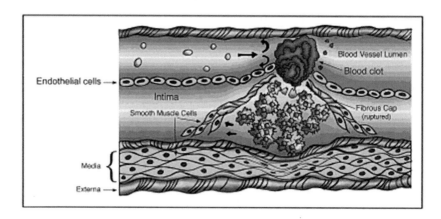

What About HDL (Good) Cholesterol?

HDL (high-density lipoprotein) can remove cholesterol from an atherosclerotic plaque and take it to the liver to be processed, thereby reducing the amount of cholesterol within the plaque. It stands to reason that having a high HDL is beneficial, and a low HDL is detrimental.

The Role of HDL:

- HDL helps to remove cholesterol from the artery wall.
- HDL has an anti-inflammatory effect.
- HDL serves as an antioxidant.
- HDL protects the endothelial lining (a thin layer of cells that line the surface of blood vessels).
- HDL helps prevent blood clots.

However, recent genetic studies have found that HDL does not necessarily correlate with heart disease risk—rather, it is how well HDL functions by removing cholesterol from the artery wall that correlates with risk. In fact, HDL can be dysfunctional and contribute to the development of atherosclerosis. Therefore, we have shifted our focus from raising HDL cholesterol to lowering LDL cholesterol and triglycerides. New medications that allow us to achieve levels of cholesterol and triglycerides that are significantly lower than before has resulted in a marked reduction in cardiovascular events, including heart attacks and strokes.

The Genesis of a Heart Attack

Proteinases released by inflammatory cells (macrophages) within the plaque break down the plaque's fibrous cap, leading to plaque rupture. When blood comes into contact with tissue factor (a clot-promoting molecule) within the plaque, a clot is formed. If the blood clot is large enough, it can completely obstruct blood flow, resulting in a heart attack.

Most plaques that rupture and cause heart attacks are not necessarily large plaques that obstruct the lumen (channel) of the artery by 80% to 90%. Instead, they are often small, inflamed plaques that may only obstruct the artery lumen by 10% to 50%. However, when a small plaque ruptures, the artery can be 100% blocked by the clot that forms in a matter of seconds. That's why most people have no prior warning. Since the root cause of this entire process is an excess number of cholesterol carrying lipoprotein particles, it stands to reason that the most effective therapy is to lower the number of these particles through lifestyle modification and medications as needed.

The National Cholesterol Education Program recommends people begin regular cholesterol testing at age twenty. There is no risk in being tested. Even if you are healthy, you should consider regular testing. Learning about your cardiovascular disease risk early will allow you to take appropriate preventive measures (e.g., dietary and exercise modification and medical therapy) that can shrink and eradicate early plaques before they become more dangerous ones that can rupture and cause heart attacks.

Key Points

> The primary cause of cardiovascular disease is an excessive number of cholesterol and triglyceride carrying atherogenic lipoproteins in the circulation that then enter the blood vessel wall and eventually lead to an atherosclerotic plaque. When these plaques rupture, a heart attack often occurs.

> Inflammation plays a major role within the atherosclerotic plaque. Proteinases produced by inflammatory cells can break down the fibrous cap of an atherosclerotic plaque. This leads to plaque rupture and heart attack.

> LDL cholesterol levels are a surrogate marker of the number of atherogenic lipoproteins.

> Soft plaques that are present early in life can shrink (regress) or be eliminated with lifestyle intervention and medical therapy before they become more dangerous, advanced plaques that can rupture and cause heart attacks.

CHAPTER 3

The Optimal Cholesterol Level

The 150 Club

You should know your cholesterol level, especially your LDL cholesterol. An optimal total cholesterol level is less than 150 mg/dl. How do we know that? Dr. William Castelli, a noted preventive cardiologist and former director of the Framingham Study, frequently mentioned the "150 club" when talking about the study results. He noted that none of the study subjects with a total cholesterol less than 150 had suffered a heart attack. It turns out that the typical American's cholesterol is far too high. In fact, a normal total cholesterol level used to be up to 300 mg/dl! Other studies supported what the Framingham Study had found—populations around the world with practically nonexistent coronary heart disease and heart attack had total cholesterol readings in the 120s to 140s. Yet today the average total cholesterol for Americans is 208 mg/dl.

Besides total cholesterol, managing your LDL cholesterol is also key to strengthening your defenses against a heart attack. Your LDL level should ideally be below 70 mg/dl for a lifetime. However, some physicians believe that LDL cholesterol should be less than 70 only if you are at very high risk and have coronary heart disease or have suffered a heart attack. That line of reasoning has never made sense to me. Why wait until you've had a heart attack to lower LDL cholesterol to levels that halt the progression of atherosclerosis or in fact reverse it? Remember, half the men and women who have a sudden heart attack have no prior warning and don't even survive their first event. Why not be proactive and lower your total cholesterol and LDL cholesterol to levels that slam the door shut on heart attacks!

Total Cholesterol Levels

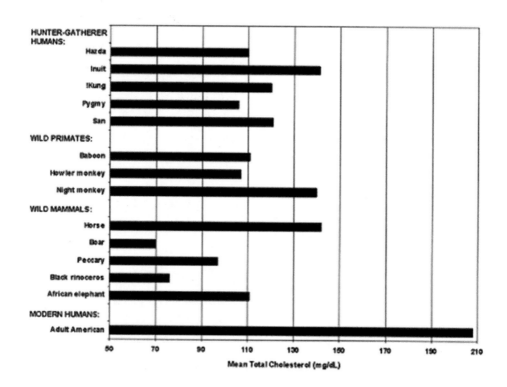

James H O'Keefe, Jr et al. JACC 2004;43:2142-2146

American College of Cardiology Foundation

What is the optimal LDL cholesterol level?

A study by James O'Keefe, M.D., and colleagues concluded that the optimal LDL cholesterol is 50 to 70 mg/dl, yet the average American has a level more than twice that amount. It is therefore no wonder that coronary heart disease and heart attacks are so prevalent.

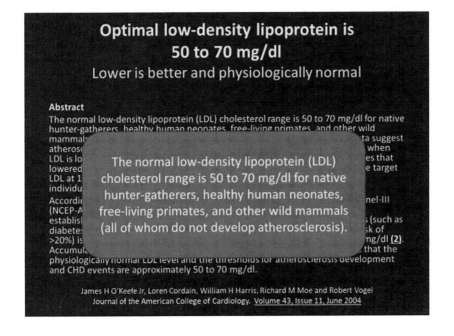

Optimal low-density lipoprotein is 50 to 70 mg/dl
Lower is better and physiologically normal

Abstract
The normal low-density lipoprotein (LDL) cholesterol range is 50 to 70 mg/dl for native hunter-gatherers, healthy human neonates, free-living primates, and other wild mammals

The normal low-density lipoprotein (LDL) cholesterol range is 50 to 70 mg/dl for native hunter-gatherers, healthy human neonates, free-living primates, and other wild mammals (all of whom do not develop atherosclerosis).

physiologically normal LDL level and the thresholds for atherosclerosis development and CHD events are approximately 50 to 70 mg/dl.

James H O'Keefe Jr, Loren Cordain, William H Harris, Richard M Moe and Robert Vogel
Journal of the American College of Cardiology. Volume 43, Issue 11, June 2004

An interesting clinical study was recently conducted with a "hunter-gatherer" population in the Bolivian Amazon. Heart attacks rarely occurred in this population, and coronary artery calcium scans to estimate the degree of coronary atherosclerosis were consistent with a very low incidence of coronary atherosclerosis (the majority had a zero-calcium score). The researchers concluded that a lifetime with low LDL cholesterol along with regular exercise, healthy nutrition with non-processed food, normal body weight, no smoking, and normal blood pressure and blood sugar could virtually eliminate coronary heart disease and heart attacks.

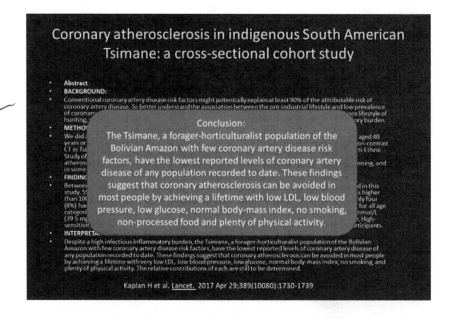

When Should We Measure Cholesterol and Begin Treatment?

It is also clear that coronary atherosclerosis begins in the young. How young? Children! Early "fatty streaks" in the arteries of children can progress to advanced plaque in late adolescence or early adulthood.

> *"Atherogenesis often begins in childhood, and some individuals begin to develop advanced plaque in late adolescence or early adulthood."*
>
> McMahan CA et al for the PDAY Group.
> Pathobiological determinants of atherosclerosis in youth risk scores are associated with early and advanced atherosclerosis.
> Pediatrics. 2006;118:1447–1455

A study looking at the coronary arteries of young soldiers in the Korean war revealed coronary atherosclerosis, including advanced plaques, were present in the majority (77%) of soldiers killed in action.

Coronary Disease Among United States Soldiers Killed in Action in Korea
Preliminary Report

- 300 autopsies
- Average age 22 years old
- 77% of hearts had evidence of coronary atherosclerosis

Enos W et al. JAMA. July 18, 1953

It is therefore abundantly clear that we have to become more proactive in our battle against heart disease. We must start in children and adolescents.

I am often asked, "Why not wait until middle age before starting treatment?" The answer is two-fold. First, if you wait that long, you can have a heart attack along the way. And second, it is much more difficult to eradicate coronary atherosclerosis later in life, as these early "soft" plaques become advanced calcified plaques.

The Risk vs Causal Exposure Paradigm: LDL as a primary cause of vascular disease

Preventing atherosclerosis before the development of significant disease is likely to be much more effective than reducing LDL when vascular disease is advanced.

Toth P et al
Journal of Clinical Lipidology
2014; 8, 594-605

Another question is how to treat the very young. It is clear that children are best treated with a healthy diet and regular exercise to control their cholesterol. Lifestyle intervention always trumps medication. As adolescents approach early adulthood, if cholesterol levels remain elevated *despite* a healthy lifestyle, then medications may be needed to achieve an optimal cholesterol level.

What about nutrition?

The top foods that have been shown to have a favorable impact on cholesterol and triglycerides are listed below.

The Top Foods to Lower Cholesterol and Triglycerides:

- Fiber-rich fruits and vegetables
- Oatmeal
- Almonds
- Beans
- Cold-water fish (salmon, tuna, sardines)
- Cinnamon
- Flaxseed
- Whole grains
- Soy protein
- Vegetable or olive oil to replace butter or margarine

The fiber contained in fruits and vegetables lowers cholesterol; in addition, plant sterols in fruits and vegetables interfere with the absorption of cholesterol. The omega-3 fatty acids in fish lower triglycerides; red wine raises "good" HDL cholesterol; and cinnamon lowers LDL cholesterol and triglycerides.

A recent study is one example of the importance of cholesterol-lowering food in our diet. Women who ate one apple a day for a year lowered their LDL cholesterol by 23% and raised their HDL cholesterol by 4%. In addition, daily apple consumption lowered inflammation and free radicals. Best of all, apple intake was associated with satiety and weight loss.

Exercise also has been shown to lower total cholesterol, raise "good" HDL cholesterol, lower triglycerides, and make the "bad" LDL cholesterol particles larger. Larger LDL particles, as previously mentioned, are less likely than smaller particles to squeeze through the artery lining, get trapped in the wall, become oxidized, and form a plaque that can eventually rupture and lead to a heart attack.

The optimal levels of cholesterol, triglycerides, lipoprotein particle number (apoB and LDL-P), and inflammation (hs-CRP):

	Recommended	Optimal
Total Cholesterol	<200 mg/dl	<150 mg/dl
LDL cholesterol	<100 mg/dl	<70 mg/dl
HDL cholesterol	>40(men) >50 (women)	>50 (men) >60(women)
Triglycerides	<150 mg/dl	<100 mg/dl
LDL-P	<1000	<700
apoB	<90 mg/dl	<70 mg/dl
hs-CRP	<2.0 mg/dl	<1.0 mg/dl

Recent research has shown that even in the presence of other major risk factors for cardiovascular disease, atherosclerosis does not seem to develop when LDL-cholesterol levels are maintained between 50mg/dl and 70 mg/dl throughout life.

The Optimal Approach to Prevent and Reverse Atherosclerosis:

- Decrease LDL cholesterol (optimal <70 mg/dl)
- Decrease triglycerides (optimal <100 mg/dl)
- Reduce vascular inflammation by achieving optimal levels of hs-CRP (<1 mg/dl)

Max and Sam

You may be asking yourself, "How does this information translate into clinical practice?" To answer this question, let's look at two different patients and how physicians may manage them with this new heart disease prevention approach.

Sam is a healthy 23-year-old who, despite healthy lifestyle choices, is unable to get his LDL cholesterol less than 100 mg/dl. He has a family history of coronary heart disease and does not want to have a heart attack in the future. Sam is placed on a statin medication and told to continue to follow a heart-healthy lifestyle. The goal is to achieve an LDL less than 70 mg/dl. Sam will continue a healthy lifestyle, and cholesterol-lowering medications will be continued as needed to maintain an optimal LDL cholesterol level.

Max is a 43-year-old who had chest pain five months ago. He underwent heart catheterization, which revealed several atherosclerotic plaques in his coronary arteries. Max was on a statin and ezetimibe, and his LDL cholesterol was 88 mg/dl. His physician continued his statin and ezetimibe and started him on a PCSK9 inhibitor to get his LDL less than 50 mg/dl to stabilize and regress (shrink) his plaques. This would make him less likely to have a future heart attack.

The above are two (of many) clinical presentations and how they may be managed if we institute a more aggressive prevention plan to avoid disastrous heart attacks in the future. Some researchers would want to conduct a randomized controlled clinical trial prior to treating LDL cholesterol in a more aggressive fashion. I would agree; a randomized clinical trial would be worthwhile. However, such a trial may last decades, and we already have clinical trial evidence that "lower is better" for LDL cholesterol. In addition, it has been shown that atherosclerotic plaques can be stabilized, reduced, or eliminated by significantly lowering LDL cholesterol. Finally, it has been established that it is safe to achieve very low levels of LDL cholesterol. So why wait? Millions of lives can be saved by being more proactive in preventing heart attacks and strokes—the time to act is now!

In conclusion, it has been well established that the primary cause of coronary heart disease is an excess number of atherogenic lipoproteins, as reflected by an elevated LDL cholesterol level. It is also clear that lower is better when it comes to LDL cholesterol—the lower we drive LDL with lifestyle intervention and pharmaceutical therapy when needed, the lower the risk of heart attack. With modern-day therapy, we have the ability to end the heart attack pandemic. We are indeed at the dawn of a new era in cardiovascular medicine.

Cholesterol Measurements

Your physician should periodically order a standard lipid profile (total cholesterol, LDL cholesterol, HDL cholesterol, and triglycerides) and achieve optimal values with lifestyle intervention and pharmaceutical therapy as needed (total cholesterol less than 150 mg/dl, LDL cholesterol less than 70 mg/dl, and triglycerides less than 150 mg/dl). Once you achieve these goals, your physician may then measure the total number of potentially bad apoB particles that can lead to atherosclerosis. If your LDL cholesterol, triglycerides, or apoB particle number is too high, then your doctor should institute further lifestyle changes and medical therapy to get you to your goal.

Is my elevated cholesterol caused by genetics or poor lifestyle?

Our cholesterol comes from two sources: what we eat and what we produce in our bodies. Some individuals have a genetic basis for their elevated cholesterol and require more aggressive medical therapy to control cholesterol and lower the risk of heart attack. Fortunately, inherited causes of high cholesterol are rare—the odds of familial heterozygous hypercholesterolemia is 1 in 250, and the odds of familial homozygous hypercholesterolemia is 1 in a million.

The overwhelming majority of men and women have elevated cholesterol levels due to a flawed lifestyle—poor dietary choices and a sedentary existence. Therefore, focus on a healthy lifestyle first with the nutritional and exercise recommendations discussed in this book—this will be sufficient for many of you to achieve optimal cholesterol and triglycerides levels. For those of you who are unable to achieve the goal despite lifestyle intervention, discuss further options with your personal physician. Your physician may decide to start pharmaceutical therapy. Remember, medications should be used if needed in addition to a healthy lifestyle, never as a substitute for a healthy lifestyle.

How Do I Know if I Have Atherosclerotic Plaques in my Arteries?

Several non-invasive methods are available to image atherosclerotic plaques in the coronary and carotid arteries. The amount of plaque in the coronary arteries is consistently associated with heart attack risk. Carotid artery intima-media thickness (a measure used to diagnose the extent of carotid artery atherosclerosis) is a well-validated test that has been shown to detect plaques in children and adults, but it is less predictive of coronary events than coronary calcium measurement with a CT scan. The optimal imaging test for evaluation of extent and quality of coronary plaques is coronary computed tomography angiography (CTA).

The latest generations of CTA scanners have high resolution for plaque and calcification and much lower radiation exposures than early generations of scanners. CTA is non-invasive and covers the entire coronary tree, and it allows evaluation of the total extent of calcified and non-calcified plaques. It is also widely available and relatively low cost. The radiation dose from the latest generation of computed tomography (CT) scanners is less than a mammogram, with an exposure of three to four mSv (millisieverts) per scan. This is less than the 6.2 mSv that the average person in the United States receives each year from natural sources like the sun. The advantage of CTA is its ability to detect non-calcified early plaques that will progress in time to an advanced calcified plaque. Early plaques are much easier to regress and eradicate with modern pharmaceutical therapy than more advanced calcified plaques. And all plaques, early soft plaques and advanced calcified plaques, are capable of rupturing, leading to a heart attack.

While CTA is presently used for unstable patients, such as those coming to the emergency room with chest pain, we may begin to use low-radiation CT scanners to detect early plaques so they can be treated and eliminated.

CTA has also emerged as the preferred choice for evaluating and characterizing composition of coronary plaques. In particular, measurement of non-calcified (low attenuation) plaque volume by CTA is a good measure of plaque burden in younger people for several reasons. Several studies demonstrate an association between non-calcified coronary plaque volume assessed by CTA and the risk of future major cardiovascular events, as well as response to statins or other preventive therapy.

One of the most interesting studies using imaging to assess progression of atherosclerosis has been with ultrasound. Studies have looked at peripheral arteries in the legs, the aorta, and the carotid arteries and found them to be a very valuable way to diagnose and follow atherosclerosis progression. Those individuals who progressed more rapidly were more likely to have heart attacks. Since ultrasound is harmless (no radiation exposure) and inexpensive, it may be the preferable approach to screen for atherosclerosis. In fact, ultrasound proved to be more predictive of heart attack risk than coronary artery calcium CT scans.

The new paradigm for eradicating atherosclerosis may include a screening ultrasound for atherosclerosis in young to middle-age adults. If they have fatty streaks or atherosclerotic plaques, then they should begin aggressive LDL cholesterol-lowering therapy to eliminate these early lesions.

The Optimal Cholesterol Level to Reverse Heart Disease

With the proper lifestyle and optimal medical therapy, it is possible to stabilize and even reverse the atherosclerotic plaques that lead to heart attacks. As we learn more about the vascular biology of atherosclerosis and the contribution of oxidation, inflammation, and immune responses to particle retention in the artery wall, we now realize that regression of atherosclerosis is an achievable goal.

Are there clinical studies that demonstrate regression or shrinking of plaques with intensive cholesterol-lowering therapy?

A plaque-regression study with the statin medication Crestor (rosuvastatin) showed just this. In 507 patients with measurable coronary artery disease, high-dose rosuvastatin significantly lowered bad (LDL) cholesterol and raised good (HDL) cholesterol that resulted in regression (decrease) in the size of the atherosclerotic plaque. The more we lower LDL cholesterol, the more plaque regression we can achieve.

Dr. K. J. Williams and colleagues published an article entitled "Rapid regression of atherosclerosis: insights from the clinical and experimental literature." They concluded that reducing LDL cholesterol levels to below 25 mg/dl has been shown to completely regress early atherosclerosis and normalize vascular function, with return of nitric oxide (a molecule that relaxes blood vessels, lowers blood pressure, reduces inflammation and decreases the risk of plaque buildup in the arteries).

Evidence for Role of Apo B Lipoproteins in Plaque Regression

Reducing LDL-C levels to below 25 mg/dL has been shown to completely regress early atheromata and normalize vascular function, with return of nitric oxide.

Williams KJ, Feig JE, Fisher EA.
Rapid regression of atherosclerosis: insights from the clinical and experimental literature.
Nat Clin Pract Cardiovasc Med. 2008;5:91–102

Another article published in the Journal Athero-sclerosis using CT angiography noted that complete plaque resolution in humans may be possible only in early stages, rather than in later stages when there is a more extensive burden of advanced calcified plaques.

Therefore, it is clear from the clinical studies that atherosclerotic plaque stabilization and regression can be achieved. In fact, with significant lowering of LDL cholesterol, complete resolution can be achieved in early stages of plaque development.

With the development of new medications that can safely lower LDL cholesterol to these very low levels, we can now eradicate early plaques and stabilize advanced plaques.

Researchers have proposed that once early plaque is eliminated with aggressive LDL cholesterol lowering to less than 50 mg/dl, the patient can then maintain an LDL cholesterol 50 mg/dl to 70 mg/dl with a healthy lifestyle and medications as needed to remain plaque free. If plaque recurs, then an intensive course of LDL cholesterol lowering can again be initiated.

An analogy to the above approach is the diagnosis and treatment of colon polyps. Gastroenterologists perform colonoscopy to identify and remove early polyps so they don't become larger and potentially cancerous. Likewise, cardiovascular imaging studies can detect atherosclerotic plaques. If detected, the patient can receive medications to significantly lower LDL cholesterol and shrink or eliminate early plaques and stabilize advanced plaques. This proactive approach will indeed lower heart attack risk.

There is also a "legacy" effect with cholesterol medications. In clinical trials with statin medications, it was noted that when the medication was stopped, there was a continued beneficial impact on heart disease risk for years. We can therefore use aggressive cholesterol-lowering therapy to stabilize and shrink coronary plaques and then shift to lifestyle intervention and moderate medical therapy as needed thereafter to maintain LDL cholesterol between 50 and 70 mg/dl to achieve a lower heart attack risk.

Legacy Effect

Primary prevention statin trials provide evidence that LDL-C lowering has a lasting impact on plaque stabilization and atherosclerotic burden and the risk of ASCVD events, or a "legacy" effect. Participants treated with statins for 3 to 5 years remains at lower cardiovascular risk over follow-up periods of 10 to 20 years.

Packard CJ, et al. New metrics needed to visualize the long-term impact of early LDL-C lowering on the cardiovascular disease trajectory. Vascul Pharmacol. 2015;71:37–39.

Key Points

> Lower is better—the lower the LDL cholesterol we can achieve with a healthy diet and medications (when needed), the lower the risk of heart attack and vascular disease.

> Earlier is better—the earlier in life we can achieve a lower LDL cholesterol, the better.

> Achieve optimal LDL cholesterol (50 mg/dl to 70 mg/dl throughout life or less than 50 mg/dl to regress or shrink existing atherosclerotic plaques.

> Non-invasive imaging techniques have allowed imaging of atherosclerotic plaques in arteries. This allows us to be aggressive with cholesterol-lowering therapy to stabilize and regress advanced plaques and potentially eradicate early plaques.

> We are now at the dawn of a new era in our quest to defeat cardiovascular disease in the United States and worldwide.

CHAPTER 4

Advances in Medical Therapy to Prevent Heart Disease

Over the past decade, we have made tremendous strides in developing medications that can stabilize and reduce blockages in our arteries. These therapeutic advances have led to a marked reduction in heart attacks and strokes. Indeed, we now have new arrows in our quiver that help us defeat this ferocious beast that we call cardiovascular disease.

New medications have been developed that enhance the lowering of LDL cholesterol, triglycerides, lipoprotein (a), and vascular inflammation. Although statin medications have been available for decades and have been shown to lower cardiovascular risk, they have not solved the heart attack pandemic. The reason for this is that statins are limited in how much they can lower LDL cholesterol. Studies have shown that statins lower heart attack risk by about 35%— well, what about the 65% who have heart attacks despite taking statin medications? This problem has been solved with the advent of new medications described below. In fact, when medications known as PCSK9 inhibitors are added to statins (with or without ezetimibe), there can be a further 50% to 60% reduction in LDL cholesterol, resulting in LDL levels that we have not been able to achieve before—levels as low as 20 mg/dl and less! Indeed, these lower levels are the reason we are able to achieve plaque regression (reduction)—and in some cases, plaque elimination!

Very high levels of triglycerides have also been a problem because they also increase heart attack risk. New medications are being developed (using a new technique called RNA therapeutics and gene silencing) that can lower triglyceride levels by 80%. In addition, a prescription-grade omega-3 fatty acid (icosapent ethyl or Vascepa), which is a highly purified EPA ethyl ester, is now available. In the landmark REDUCE-IT trial, this medication was used in patients at high cardiovascular risk who were already taking optimal statin therapy for LDL cholesterol control but had residual elevation of triglycerides—the net result was a highly significant lowering of major adverse cardiovascular events by 25%.

Lastly, genetic research has paved the way for medications that can be used for conditions other than elevated LDL cholesterol and triglycerides. For instance, lipoprotein(a), a highly atherogenic particle, is present in 20% of the population, and it often leads to premature heart attacks and death. Previously, there has been no medication that could significantly lower elevated lipoprotein

(a) and reduce heart attack risk. Now we have a pharmaceutical agent described below that can significantly and safely lower lipoprotein (a) by 80%. Clinical outcome trials are now underway to see if this profound lowering of elevated lipo-protein (a) will result in a significant reduction in heart attack risk. This can truly be a game changer.

The medications that are presently available and those that are very promising in clinical trials are summarized below.

- **Statins**
  Statins reduce cholesterol production and have become the first-line medication to lower cho-lesterol. They have been shown very safe and effective in lowering LDL cholesterol. Most impor-tantly, numerous clinical trials have demon-strated a significant reduction in heart attack risk in patients with elevated LDL cholesterol. Popular brands include Crestor (rosuvastatin), Lipitor (atorvastatin) and Zocor (simvastatin). Since they are available as generics, they are very cost effective.

- **Ezetimibe (Zetia)**
  Ezetimibe is a cholesterol-absorption inhibitor and has been shown to be safe and effective as monotherapy and when used in combination with statin medication. The IMPROVE-IT trial demonstrated safety and efficacy of ezetimibe

as well as a further reduction in cardiovascular risk when added to statin medications.

- **Resins**

  Resins such as colesevelam (Welchol) are bile acid—binding resins. They work by removing bile acid from the body, which causes the liver to make more bile acid by using cholesterol, thereby lowering cholesterol levels in the blood. They have become less popular due to compliance issues and their tendency to raise triglyceride levels.

- **Fibrates**

  Fibrates, such as fenofibrate, can lower triglyceride levels. The PROMINENT trial will determine if lowering elevated triglycerides with pemafibrate in diabetics will improve clinical outcome.

- **PCSK9 Inhibitors**

  PCSK9 is a protein produced in the liver and released into the circulation, where it can bind to an LDL receptor on the surface of the liver. The LDL receptor-PCSK9 complex is then carried into the liver, where it is metabolized. This results in a decrease in LDL receptors on the liver surface, which in turn leads to fewer receptors to remove LDL cholesterol particles from circulation, resulting in an increase in LDL cholesterol levels. Monoclonal antibodies were developed to target and inhibit PCSK9, thereby lowering LDL cholesterol. Clinical trials have demonstrated a significant lowering of LDL cholesterol levels by 50% on top of statins. Most importantly, PCSK9 clinical outcome trials (Fourier and Odyssey Outcomes) have shown a significant reduction in cardiovascular events. Repatha (evolocumab) and Praluent (alirocumab) are PCSK9 inhibitors approved for use in the United States, and they are given by subcutaneous injection every two to four weeks.

- **Icosapent Ethyl (Vascepa)**
  Icosapent ethyl is a highly purified EPA ethyl ester (omega-3 fatty acid) that lowers triglycerides and has a number of beneficial actions that lower heart attack risk. The REDUCE-IT trial showed that icosapent ethyl lowered cardiovascular risk by 25% when added to optimal statin therapy in high-risk patients with residual triglyceride elevation.
- **Mipomersen**
  Used for patients with high cholesterol with the genetic disorder familial hypercholesterolemia (FH).
- **Lomitapide**
  Used for patients with high cholesterol with the genetic disorder familial hypercholesterolemia (FH).
- **Inclisiran**
  Inclisiran is a drug that interferes with the production of PCSK9 in the liver. It is given by subcutaneous injection every six months and

has been shown to be safe and effective in lowering LDL cholesterol. In fact, inclisiran has been shown to lower LDL cholesterol by 50% when added to statin therapy. A clinical outcome trial is underway (ORION 4). This medication may indeed be a game changer since it only needs to be given twice per year, and it has been shown to be highly effective in lowering LDL cholesterol.

- **Bempedoic Acid**

  Bempedoic Acid is similar to statins in that it inhibits production of cholesterol in the liver at a site just proximal to where statins work. It has been shown to further reduce cholesterol when added to statins and ezetimibe.

- **Lipoprotein(a) gene silencing**

  Lipoprotein(a) is a particle that is elevated in 20% of the population and can cause premature heart attacks, blood clots, and calcific aortic stenosis. The gene for lipoprotein(a) is inherited, and the levels are not lowered by diet, exercise, or statin therapy. A new technique called antisense technology is a way to block production of lipoprotein(a) within the cell and thereby lower levels of this lipoprotein by 80%. A clinical outcome trial is underway (Lp(a) HORIZON), and hopefully it will significantly lower cardiovascular risk in patients with elevated levels of lipoprotein(a).

- **Apolipoprotein C3 silencing**
Apolipoprotein C3 (APO C3) is a protein that elevates triglyceride levels and thereby increases heart attack risk. Studies have shown that an antisense therapeutic approach can lower apolipoprotein C3 levels by nearly 80%. A clinical outcome study is underway to determine if this new approach will lower cardiovascular events in patients with elevated triglyceride levels.

Is it safe to achieve very low levels of LDL cholesterol?

With lifestyle intervention and advances in pharmaceutical therapy, we are now able to achieve very low levels of LDL cholesterol that heretofore we have not been able to achieve. These levels, as low as single digits, have allowed us to stabilize, regress, and in some cases, eradicate atherosclerotic plaques. This more aggressive approach to LDL reduction has led to a significant reduction in heart attacks, strokes, and cardiovascular death. But what about safety? Is it safe to dramatically reduce LDL, and isn't cholesterol needed for normal cellular function? These questions and concerns have been answered by clinical trials addressing safety.

Scientific studies have shown that all tissues in our body are capable of making cholesterol and therefore do not need dietary cholesterol for their physiologic needs.

> *"All tissues are capable of synthesizing enough cholesterol to meet their metabolic and structural needs. Consequently, there is no evidence for a biological requirement for dietary cholesterol."*
>
> *Dietary DRI Reference Intakes. The Essential Guide to Nutrient Requirements. Institute of Medicine of the National Academies. The National Academies Press, Washington, DC.*

Studies have also looked at individuals with rare inherited disorders who were born with very low cholesterol levels due to their genetics. These men and women have been able to lead normal and healthy lives with very low risk of cardiovascular disease. In addition, there was no evidence of harm caused by their very low LDL cholesterol levels.

> ## The Risk vs Causal Exposure Paradigm: LDL as a primary cause of vascular disease
>
> *"Clinical studies of individuals genetically predisposed to modestly lower LDL-C over a lifetime results in a much greater reduction in CVD."*
>
> *Toth P et al*
> *Journal of Clinical Lipidology*
> *2014; 8, 594-605*

Numerous statin trials have found no significant safety issues with LDL cholesterol lowering.

The IMPROVE-IT trial looked at the addition of ezetimibe, a medication that inhibits the absorption of cholesterol from the gastrointestinal tract, to the statin medication simvastatin. This combination further lowered LDL cholesterol from the high 60s to the low 50s and resulted in a significant reduction in major adverse cardiovascular events. Best of all, there were no adverse safety signals observed.

One of the more recent and exciting medications that has been developed to lower LDL cholesterol are PCSK9-inhibitors. PCSK9 is a protein that decreases amount of LDL cholesterol that can be removed from the bloodstream by the liver. By inhibiting PCSK9, LDL cholesterol is significantly lowered. The FOURIER trial evaluated evolocumab, a PCK9-inhibitor, on a background of statin therapy. LDL cholesterol levels were lowered to a median of 30 mg/dl, and the risk of cardiovascular events were reduced. Importantly, there was no significant adverse effects of the medication.

The ODYSSEY OUTCOMES trial evaluated high-risk patients with a prior heart attack who were receiving high-intensity statin therapy. They found that the risk of recurrent cardiovascular events was lower among those who received the PSCK9-inhibitor alirocumab than among those who received placebo, and there were no significant safety issues. LDL cholesterol levels were reduced to as low as 38mg/dl in the statin/alirocumab group.

The ORION 1 trial examined the efficacy and safety of inclisiran, a molecule that interferes with the production of PCSK9 in the liver. When added to statin therapy in high-risk individuals, inclisiran significantly lowered LDL cholesterol (66% of patients had an LDL less than 25 mg/dl six months after a single subcutaneous injection). No significant adverse events were observed in those receiving inclisiran compared to placebo.

Key Points

> With lifestyle intervention and advances in pharmaceutical therapy, we are now able to safely achieve very low levels of LDL cholesterol that heretofore we have not been able to achieve. These levels, as low as single digits, have allowed us to stabilize, regress, and in some cases, eradicate atherosclerotic plaques.

> New medications have also been developed that lower triglycerides, lipoprotein(a), and vascular inflammation. These metabolic risk factors contribute to cardiovascular disease; therefore, reducing them lowers heart attack risk.

> REDUCE-IT, a landmark clinical trial, demonstrated that lowering triglycerides with the omega-3 icosapent ethyl in patients at high cardiovascular-disease risk who had optimal LDL cholesterol levels significantly lowered major adverse cardiovascular events (including heart attacks and strokes).

> Inclisiran is a new medication that may indeed be a game changer since it only needs to be given twice per year, and it has been shown to be safe and highly effective in lowering LDL cholesterol.

CHAPTER 5

Blood Tests to Uncover Hidden Cardiovascular Risk

Blood tests are a useful way of detecting problems that may not be apparent. They are also essential to effectively monitor already-diagnosed conditions and to ensure that medical treatment and lifestyle changes are working.

When I do blood tests for my new patients, in addition to a CBC, chemistry panel, and standard lipid profile, I test for the number of cholesterol-carrying particles (apoB), high-sensitivity CRP (hs-CRP), and lipoprotein(a) (LP(a)). The tests described below are important for uncovering hidden risk for heart attack, stroke, and vascular disease, thereby allowing physicians to individualize treatment programs that will best lower their patients' risk of disability and death from cardiovascular disease.

Routine CBC

• What is it? A Complete Blood Count is one of the most common tests performed. It measures your red and white blood cell count, platelet count, hemoglobin, and hematocrit levels.

- Why you need it: a CBC can detect if you are anemic, dehydrated, have an infection or blood-based cancer, and measures your platelet count.

Chemistry panel

- What is it? A chemistry panel assesses factors in the blood, such as blood glucose; electrolytes, such as calcium, potassium, and sodium; kidney function (blood urea nitrogen and creatinine); and liver function (such as transaminase levels and bilirubin).
- Why you need it: a chemistry panel can determine if you have diabetes, how well your kidneys and liver are functioning, and if you may have other important metabolic disorders.

Thyroid function panel

- What is it? Your thyroid gland, along with the pituitary gland, produces hormones that regulate your body's metabolism. This test measures TSH (thyroid stimulating hormone), T3, and T4.
- Why you need it: this test can identify thyroid disorders (hyperthyroid, hypothyroid) that can cause weight gain or loss, as well as impact the heart and other organs.

Lipid profile

- What is it? This is the traditional group of tests that measure your cholesterol and triglyceride levels. A basic lipid profile will include total

cholesterol, high-density lipoprotein (HDL) cholesterol, low-density lipoprotein (LDL) cholesterol, and triglycerides.
- Why you need it: these test results allow you to assess and monitor your risk for heart attack, stroke, and vascular disease.

hs-CRP

- What is it? This test measures the levels of high-sensitivity C-reactive protein (hs-CRP), which rise in response to vascular inflammation.
- Why you need it: Damage to your arteries from plaques and fatty deposits will produce an inflammatory response, with corresponding increased levels of hs-CRP. Remember, atherosclerosis is, in part, a chronic inflammatory disease, and hs-CRP is a marker of vascular inflammation. If hs-CRP is elevated, your risk of a heart attack or stroke is increased. Therefore, knowing your levels can help you and your doctor assess your cardiovascular risk.

Apo B

- What is it? ApoB (apolipoprotein-B) is a protein that is attached to atherogenic (potentially harmful) lipoproteins, such as LDL (low-density lipoprotein). There is one apoB protein for each atherogenic particle like LDL. Therefore, apoB is a measure of the number of potentially harmful atherogenic particles and is a better predictor of heart attack risk than cholesterol.

- Why you need it: This test measures the number of potentially harmful atherogenic particles that can enter the wall of the blood vessel and cause the plaque buildup—which leads to a heart attack. High levels of apoB have been shown to be a better predictor of heart attack risk than the LDL cholesterol.

Lp(a)

- Lp(a) or lipoprotein(a) is an LDL particle with an apoA protein attachment that makes it particularly atherogenic (harmful). It is associated with an increased risk of heart attack, stroke, and thrombosis (blood clot).
- Why you may need it: High Lp(a) levels are inherited and predictive of heart attack and stroke as well as thrombosis. In addition, it also increases the risk of calcific aortic stenosis.

Atherogenesis, or the development of plaques, is the result of an increased flux of apoB lipoproteins, like LDL, *into* the artery wall, along with retention of these particles so they can't leave. Atherosclerosis cannot develop when particle number (measured by apoB) is low. That means your goal is to keep apoB levels in the optimal range.

The optimal total cholesterol level is less than 150 mg/dl. Yet on average, Americans have a total cholesterol of about 208 mg/dl. Your LDL cholesterol level should ideally be at or below 70 mg/dl; however, the average LDL cholesterol in America is 116 mg/dl.

OPTIMAL CHOLESTEROL and TRIGLYCERIDES	
Total Cholesterol Goal:	<150 mg/dl
LDL Cholesterol Goal:	<70 mg/dl
Triglyceride Goal:	<100 mg/dl

Key Points

> Blood tests are important to identify metabolic derangements in our body so that we can correct them with lifestyle intervention and pharmaceutical therapy if needed.

> Routine blood tests include a complete blood count (CBC), chemistry panel (e.g., electrolytes, kidney function, liver function), and lipid panel (total cholesterol, HDL cholesterol, LDL cholesterol, and triglycerides).

> ApoB (apolipoprotein-B) measures the total number of particles that can lead to plaque formation and heart attacks.

➢ Lp(a) or lipoprotein(a) is an atherogenic (potentially harmful) particle that increases the risk of heart attack, stroke, and thrombosis (blood clot).

➢ hs-CRP (high-sensitivity C-reactive protein) is a marker of vascular inflammation. If elevated, it can be lowered with lifestyle intervention and medications if needed.

➢ Thyroid function panel (T3, T4 and TSH) can detect an overactive or underactive thyroid gland. Hypothyroidism (underactive thyroid) can lead to high cholesterol and an increased risk of heart attack. Hyperthyroidism (overactive thyroid) can lead to rapid heartbeat and atrial fibrillation and increase the risk of stroke.

CHAPTER 6

Optimal Nutrition for Health and Longevity

"Let food be thy medicine . . . "
—Hippocrates, 400 BC

Since healthy nutrition is such a key component to a heart-healthy life, I have devoted an entire chapter to this topic. I will discuss all aspects of nutrition, including a dietary plan for long-term health, as well as a sensible approach to shed those extra pounds and achieve ideal body weight.

So first things first. What is your weight? Do you feel it is optimal? Have you been carrying around an extra 10, 20, or 50 pounds that you wish you could shed? Living with extra fat and being overweight or obese are known risk factors for not only a heart attack and stroke but a multitude of other disease states, including diabetes, cancer, and osteoarthritis.

But sometimes weight doesn't tell the entire story, which is why the medical community also relies on a metric called the Body Mass Index (BMI). When physicians and researchers discuss statistics of how many people in this country are overweight or obese, they are based on the BMI.

Body Mass Index (BMI)

The BMI uses your weight plus your height to assess your body fat. BMI is a number obtained by first taking one's weight in pounds and dividing it by the square of his or her height in inches. Then multiply that by 703. Since it is a rather complicated formula, there are many online calculators to figure out your BMI, and I also have provided a handy chart below to help you figure yours.

Body Mass Index:

Weight in Pounds

Height	100	110	120	130	140	150	160	170	180	190	200	210	220	230	240	250
4'	30.5	33.6	36.6	39.7	42.7	45.8	48.8	51.9	54.9	58.0	61.0	64.1	67.1	70.2	73.2	76.3
4'2"	28.1	30.9	33.7	36.6	39.4	42.2	45.0	47.8	50.6	53.4	56.2	59.1	61.9	64.7	67.5	70.3
4'4"	26.0	28.6	31.2	33.8	36.4	39.0	41.6	44.2	46.8	49.4	52.0	54.6	57.2	59.8	62.4	65.0
4'6"	24.1	26.5	28.9	31.3	33.8	36.2	38.6	41.0	43.4	45.8	48.2	50.6	53.0	55.4	57.9	60.3
4'8"	22.4	24.7	26.9	29.1	31.4	33.6	35.9	38.1	40.4	42.6	44.8	47.1	49.3	51.6	53.8	56.0
4'10"	20.9	23.0	25.1	27.2	29.3	31.3	33.4	35.5	37.6	39.7	41.8	43.9	46.0	48.1	50.2	52.2
5'	19.5	21.5	23.4	25.4	27.3	29.3	31.2	33.2	35.2	37.1	39.1	41.0	43.0	44.9	46.9	48.8
5'2"	18.3	20.1	21.9	23.8	25.6	27.4	29.3	31.1	32.9	34.7	36.6	38.4	40.2	42.1	43.9	45.7
5'4"	17.2	18.9	20.6	22.3	24.0	25.7	27.5	29.2	30.9	32.6	34.3	36.0	37.8	39.5	41.2	42.9
5'6"	16.1	17.8	19.4	21.0	22.6	24.2	25.8	27.4	29.0	30.7	32.3	33.9	35.5	37.1	38.7	40.3
5'8"	15.2	16.7	18.2	19.8	21.3	22.8	24.3	25.8	27.4	28.9	30.4	31.9	33.4	35.0	36.5	38.0
5'10"	14.3	15.8	17.2	18.7	20.1	21.5	23.0	24.4	25.8	27.3	28.7	30.1	31.6	33.0	34.4	35.9
6'	13.6	14.9	16.3	17.6	19.0	20.3	21.7	23.1	24.4	25.8	27.1	28.5	29.8	31.2	32.5	33.9
6'2"	12.8	14.1	15.4	16.7	18.0	19.3	20.5	21.8	23.1	24.4	25.7	27.0	28.2	29.5	30.8	32.1
6'4"	12.2	13.4	14.6	15.8	17.0	18.3	19.5	20.7	21.9	23.1	24.3	25.6	26.8	28.0	29.2	30.4
6'6"	11.6	12.7	13.9	15.0	16.2	17.3	18.5	19.6	20.8	22.0	23.1	24.3	25.4	26.6	27.7	28.9
6'8"	11.0	12.1	13.2	14.3	15.4	16.5	17.6	18.7	19.8	20.9	22.0	23.1	24.2	25.3	26.4	27.5
6'10"	10.5	11.5	12.5	13.6	14.6	15.7	16.7	17.8	18.8	19.9	20.9	22.0	23.0	24.0	25.1	26.1
7'	10.0	11.0	12.0	13.0	13.9	14.9	15.9	16.9	17.9	18.9	19.9	20.9	21.9	22.9	23.9	24.9

Height in Feet and Inches

http://www.freebmicalculator.net

Underweight   Nomal   Overweight   Obesity

The benefit of the BMI is that it standardizes the risk based on both height and weight. A BMI of 18.5–24.9 is considered normal, while a BMI of 25–29.9 is overweight. A BMI of 30 or greater indicates the individual is obese.

More than 60 percent of the U.S. population is overweight or obese. That's right. Almost one in three people are at significantly greater risk for cardiovascular disease and a number of other diseases based on their BMI. And as more and more adults become bigger and heavier, so too are our children becoming overweight and obese at an alarming rate. According to the CDC, childhood obesity has tripled over the last thirty years. Approximately 19% of children and adolescents 19 and younger are obese. It is a sad statistic—but one we can prevent.

Culprit of Obesity–The Toxic American Diet and Lifestyle

Most people are well aware that obesity is far more common today than it was just a few decades ago. The United States has one of the highest rates of obesity in the world. It's commonly accepted that one-third of adults are obese.

Maintaining a healthy weight is important for many aspects of health, but excess weight has particular implications for cardiovascular health. Besides increasing the risk of heart attack and stroke, obesity also increases the risk of:

- Hypertension
- Type 2 diabetes
- Abnormal cholesterol and triglycerides levels
- Cancer
- Gallbladder disease

- Sleep apnea syndrome
- Osteoarthritis

What you eat is the single most important factor in your health. And our diet is killing us.

Part of the problem is what our typical American diet doesn't include—not enough fresh fruits, vegetables, and whole grains. Instead, we have replaced these naturally available food sources with highly processed foods that are injurious to our health.

Children at Risk

Research is showing alarming statistics about children with cardiovascular disease manifesting as fatty streaks, the earliest stage of atherosclerosis, in their arteries. In a population-based sample of 5-to-17-year-olds, 70% of obese youth had at least one risk factor for cardiovascular disease.

It doesn't take much to see that overweight and obese children will become overweight and obese adults, making them a ticking time bomb for a heart attack.

Our Children Are at Risk!

Seeing youngsters with signs of cardiovascular disease and atherosclerosis is very *disheartening*. For baby boomers with heart disease, it is plausible that we just didn't know the dangers of processed foods, sedentary lifestyles, or high LDL cholesterol. But today we do! An elevated level of cholesterol is much more dangerous when established early in life than if established in later years. Unfortunately, today's children are the first generation ever who many authorities predict will not live as long as their parents. Your goal is to not only help yourself become healthy but optimize the health of your children and grandchildren so that they become protected as well.

Face the Scales

When thinking about losing weight, it truly is a matter of avoiding processed or refined food and being aware of calories taken in versus calories burned. Numerically, 3,500 calories burned equals one pound of weight lost. This is why it is so important to stay active and choose your calories carefully. Choosing highly processed, calorie-dense and nutrient-depleted food is doing your body a big disservice. You wouldn't put diesel fuel in your gasoline-powered car, so why would you put the wrong food in your body? The wrong fuel in your car results in a breakdown of your vehicle and costly repairs. The wrong food in your body leads to disease and even costlier treatment!

Be Realistic and Succeed!

When trying to lose weight, I will say to you what I say to my patients. Be patient and be realistic.

You cannot lose 20 pounds in 2 weeks, and if you could, it wouldn't be healthy. Achieving a healthy weight is about a lifestyle change—eating the right foods and staying physically active. Avoid sugar, refined starches, saturated fat, and trans fat. Select fiber-rich foods with a low glycemic index. A Mediterranean diet is one of the best examples of a healthy diet for a lifetime that leads to weight control and long-term health.

The Mediterranean diet: a cultural model for healthy eating:

- Plant foods (fruit, vegetables, whole grains, beans, nuts, and seeds)
- Fresh fruit as the typical daily dessert
- Olive oil as the principal source of fat
- Dairy products (principally cheese and yogurt)
- Fish and poultry consumed in moderate amounts
- Eggs (zero to four) consumed weekly
- Red meat consumed in low amounts
- Low in saturated fat (<7% of energy), with total fat ranging from <25% to >35% of energy

Willett WC et al. AM J Clin Nutr. 1995 Jun;61:1402S–1406S.

Try to lose one-to-two pounds per week. This may sound very modest, but it is an achievable goal and can lead to 50-to-100-pound weight loss over a year! For those of you who need to lose this much weight to reach a normal BMI, this can be accomplished and maintained for a lifetime.

To shed one pound means you must burn (or eliminate) an extra 3,500 calories per week, or 500 calories per day. This can be achieved. One sugar sweetened soda contains 150 calories. A perfect example of a way to reduce 500 calories per day would be to cut out two sodas and walk for approximately 30 to 45 minutes per day.

Fiber–The Key to Weight Control

Fiber-rich foods are very important for optimal health and weight control. Sadly, the highly processed food we consume is deficient in soluble and insoluble fiber—and we pay the price for this!

How much fiber should we consume? On average, American adults eat only 10 grams of total fiber per day, while the United States Department of Agriculture's recommended daily amount for adults up to age fifty is 25 grams/day for women and 38 grams/day for men. Women and men older than fifty should have 20 and 30 daily grams, respectively.

What are the health benefits of a fiber-rich diet? Below are listed ten important reasons to consume an adequate amount of fiber.

1. Weight Control

A study in the *Annals of Internal Medicine* found that even if increasing your fiber intake is the only dietary change you make, you will still lose weight. Dieters who were told to get at least 30 grams of fiber a day, but given no other dietary parameters, lost a significant amount of weight. In fact, they lost nearly as much as a group put on a much more complex diet that required limiting calories and curtailing various food groups. Fiber-rich foods not only fill you up faster and keep you satisfied longer, but they also prevent your body from absorbing some of the calories in the foods you eat. Fiber binds with fat and sugar molecules as they travel through the GI (gastrointestinal) tract, thereby lowering the number of calories you actually get.

2. Maintain a Healthier Weight Over Time

Fiber consumption can also help you avoid putting pounds back on. Research has shown that men and women who consume more fiber tend to be leaner than those who consume less. Fiber intake leads to satiety or feeling of fullness—this suppresses your appetite, and you eat and snack less.

3. Type 2 Diabetes Risk

Recent research has found that people who ate the most fiber (>26 grams a day) lowered their risk of type 2 diabetes by 18%. The researchers noted that keeping blood sugar levels controlled and maintaining a healthy weight may help stave off the development of diabetes.

4. Lower Heart Disease Risk

A study published in the *British Medical Journal* found that fiber intake significantly lowered heart disease risk. That's partly due to fiber's ability to lower cholesterol levels by decreasing absorption in the GI tract. Other studies have shown that fiber consumption lowers the risk of heart attacks by:

- Lowering serum LDL cholesterol
- Reducing lipid peroxidation
- Improving insulin sensitivity
- Weight control and reduced incidence of obesity and metabolic syndrome
- Beneficial impact on gut flora

It also has been reported that heart attack survivors who ate the most fiber had a 25% reduction in overall mortality over nine years. Every increase of 10 grams of fiber each day was linked to a 15% lower risk of dying over the study period.

5. Healthier Gut Bacteria

The good bacteria that make up your microbiome feed off fiber. As your gut bacteria consume fiber that has fermented in your gastrointestinal tract, they produce short-chain fatty acids that have a host of benefits—including lowering systemic inflammation. A recent Italian study found that eating a high-fiber Mediterranean diet was associated with higher levels of healthy short-chain fatty acids.

6. Reduce Your Risk of Cancer

Every 10 grams of fiber you eat is associated with a 10% reduced risk of colorectal cancer and a 5% fall in breast cancer risk, according to a study published in the *Annals of Oncology*.

7. Live Longer, Period

Researchers at the Harvard School of Public Health recently found that people who often ate fiber-rich cereals and whole grains had a 19% and 17%, respectively, reduced risk of death—from any cause—compared to those who consumed less fiber.

8. Avoid Constipation

9. Get an All-Natural Detox

Fiber naturally promotes the elimination of toxins from your gastrointestinal tract. Soluble fiber traps potentially harmful compounds and limits the amount of time that chemicals like BPA, mercury, and pesticides stay in your system. The faster they go through you, the less chance they have to cause harm.

10. Healthier Bones

Soluble fiber found in asparagus, leeks, soybeans, wheat, and oats have been shown to increase the bioavailability of minerals like calcium in the foods you eat, which may help maintain bone density.

What foods are fiber rich?

Fruits and vegetables, whole grains, beans and legumes, and nuts are all fiber rich. These foods are all part of a healthy Mediterranean diet, truly a high-fiber diet.

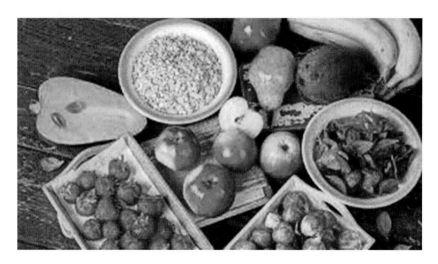

The Glycemic Index and Weight Control

In addition to a fiber-rich diet, knowledge of the glycemic index can help you lose weight and control your blood sugar. Fiber-rich foods generally have a low glycemic index.

What is the glycemic index? The glycemic index is a relative ranking of carbohydrate in foods according to how they affect blood glucose levels. It is a value assigned to foods based on how slowly or how quickly those foods cause increases in blood glucose levels. Foods low on the glycemic index scale tend to release glucose slowly and steadily. Foods high on the glycemic index release glucose rapidly. Pure glucose is given the value of one hundred, which represents the relative rise in the blood glucose level of consuming glucose in two hours. For those interested in losing weight or maintaining the weight they lost, avoiding foods with a high glycemic index is advised. Carbohydrates with a low glycemic index value (55 or less) are more slowly digested, absorbed, and metabolized, and cause a lower and slower rise in blood glucose and, therefore, insulin levels. This helps to improve satiety, lower the risk of insulin resistance and diabetes, and control body weight.

Glycemic Index
Low: 55 or less
Moderate: 56–69
High: 70 or greater

Below is a ranking of various foods and their glycemic index.

Low Glycemic Index:

Low-Glycemic Fruit

- Apples
- Dried apricots
- Under-ripe banana

- Peaches
- Strawberries
- Oranges
- Cherries
- Coconut
- Cranberries
- Blueberries
- Pears
- Plums
- Grapefruit

Low-Glycemic Vegetables

- Carrots
- Green peas
- Onions
- Lettuce
- Greens (spinach, kale, collards, beet)
- Green beans
- Tomatoes
- Cucumbers
- Bok choy
- Mushrooms
- Artichokes
- Brussels sprouts
- Cabbage
- Broccoli
- Cauliflower
- Celery
- Eggplant
- Peppers (bell peppers, jalapenos, serrano, etc.)

- Zucchini and crookneck squash
- Snow peas

Low-Glycemic Grains

- Barley
- Whole wheat kernels
- All-Bran and Fiber One cereals
- Oat bran and rice bran cereals
- Whole grain pasta
- Lasagna with meat and/or cheese, ravioli, tortellini, and other stuffed pasta
- Whole grain pumpernickel bread
- Sourdough bread
- Wheat tortilla

High Glycemic Index:

- Watermelon (72)
- Honey (73)
- Doughnuts (75)
- French fries (76)
- White rice (89)
- Certain cereals (76)
- Millet (71)
- White bread (71)
- Pumpkin (75)
- Instant oatmeal (83)
- Rice pasta (78)
- Parsnips (97)
- Corn syrup (73)
- Table sugar (75)

- Soda (74)
- Puffed rice (78)

To achieve optimal weight and health:

- Choose healthy carbohydrates that are fiber rich.
- Include plant-based proteins, as well as fish and chicken and healthy fats found in nuts, seeds, and avocados.
- Avoid high-glycemic-index foods.
- Avoid sugar and refined starches.
- Daily physical activity

The Bathroom Scale

I doubt that you ever ran out of gas while driving your car because you forgot to look at the fuel gauge. Yet most of you forget to look at the "fuel gauge" for your body—the scale in your bathroom. If you are overweight or obese, weigh yourself daily and strive for one to two pounds of weight loss per week. If you don't achieve this goal, you have one of three choices:

1: Eat less
2: Exercise more
3: Eat less and exercise more

Eating less does not mean that you walk around hungry. Remember, staples of the Mediterranean diet include fruits, vegetables, beans, and nuts—foods that are rich in fiber that lead to satiety.

> Be smart—don't try to lose a large amount of weight in a short period of time. This is usually associated with fluid and electrolyte loss, leading to dehydration—this is not healthy and can lead to serious side effects, like heart rhythm disturbances and kidney malfunction.

Highly Processed Foods

Many processed foods widely available in our supermarkets, grocery stores, and fast-food restaurants have been stripped of their key healthful ingredients and pumped full of artificial preservatives. Moreover, our food contains an excessive amount of unhealthy fats, refined sugar, and sodium.

Many of you know these foods are bad, but you resist change. I will show you how a Mediterranean diet is easy to prepare, delicious, and will lead to weight control and optimal health.

Fruit Juice?

No thanks! Converting whole fruit to juice eliminates much of the healthy fiber and nutrients.

Fat: The Good, Bad, and Ugly

There are three types of fat in our diet: unsaturated fat (good), saturated fat (bad), and trans fat (just plain ugly). Unsaturated fats (monounsaturated and polyunsaturated fats) are healthy fats. When you look at a food nutritional label, you will see a breakdown of the fats to help you know how healthy or unhealthy a food is.

Saturated fats are unhealthy fats. They raise "bad" LDL cholesterol and increase the risk of heart attack and cancer. They are found in animal products, such as red meat, lard, butter, milk, cheese, and certain tropical oils like palm and coconut oil.

Trans fatty acids, or trans fats, are the most unhealthy fats. They are "manufactured" fat born out of an evolving need for more efficient foods that can withstand long shelf lives. Trans fats are manufactured by taking oils—mainly vegetable oils—and putting them through a process called hydrogenation. Trans fats are found in many sweet, savory, and processed foods such as margarine, French fries, potato chips, cookies, crackers, baked goods, and pastries, and certain frozen foods—most of which can sit in your cupboard for many months without going rancid.

While scientists may have succeeded in making the foods last longer, they couldn't have created foods worse for our health. They raise "bad" LDL cholesterol, lower "good" HDL cholesterol, increase inflammation in the body, and make blood clots more likely to form.

Know Your Fats

Unsaturated (good)	Fish oil, nuts
Saturated (bad)	Butter, meat, cheese
Trans Fats (plain ugly)	Packaged cookies, chips, pastries

Trans-fat consumption has been linked to heart disease, cancer, Alzheimer's disease, and diabetes. It has been found to be so harmful that certain countries, like Denmark, have banned the use of them more than two decades ago. The Food and Drug Administration (FDA) has recently banned trans fats in the United States.

Common Foods That Contain Trans Fat

Cookies	Doughnuts
Cake mixes	Margarine
Candy	French fries
Chips	Vegetable shortening
Crackers	Coffee creamers

A note of consumer caution!

Beware of the trans-fat hoax: Food companies are allowed to list zero trans fat on their label and still have up to 500 mg of trans fat per serving. Imagine if five of your daily foods have this amount. You are consuming 2,500 mg of trans fat in one day. This can result in a significant amount of trans fat consumption per week. Read the food label—if it lists trans fats or partially hydrogenated oil, don't eat it!

High-Fructose Corn Syrup

Most of us know to avoid excess sugar, whether that's table sugar, candies, or syrups. But there's an even more sinister sweetener lurking on your shelves: high-fructose corn syrup. This sweetener is a favorite of the food industry since it is sweeter than ordinary table sugar, is inexpensive, and prolongs the shelf life of food. It is found in many beverages and foods, including soft drinks, sports drinks, packaged cookies, and other baked goods.

The real danger posed by high-fructose corn syrup, however, is the metabolic havoc it causes. In contrast to ordinary sugar, high-fructose corn syrup is not utilized by the muscles as an energy source. Instead, it goes directly to the liver, where it spikes triglyceride production, a major risk factor for heart disease.

Apparently, that is not all. Research has shown that people who ate or drank more than 74 grams per day of fructose (the equivalent of only 2.5 sugary soft drinks per day) increased their risk of developing high blood pressure or hypertension. A normal blood pressure reading is below 120/80 mmHg. But consuming more than 74 grams of fructose per day led to a 28%, 36%, and 87% higher risk for blood pressure levels of 135/85, 140/90, and 160/100 mmHg, respectively, in a study population of 4,528 adults 18 years of age or older with no prior history of hypertension.

Coincidence? High-Fructose Corn Syrup and Obesity

Since its introduction in 1970, the amount of high-fructose corn syrup in our food has steadily increased; currently, the average American consumes about 75 pounds of this sweetener each year. Our obesity rate also jumped from 15% to 30% during the same period, which many nutritionists believe is not a coincidence.

My Beef with Beef

Americans eat too much red meat. If you eat five ounces of red meat more than once a week, you are one of them. Research study after research study has shown that red meat is bad for our health, yet we skirt around the issue and downplay the serious health consequences of eating it. It seems we are obsessed with red meat. We have bacon for breakfast, a hamburger or hot dog for lunch, and steak or meatloaf for dinner! Gourmet hamburger restaurants are the rage, and extensive commercial marketing campaigns have been launched to support continued consumption.

So What's Wrong with Meat?

Red meat is high in saturated fats, which raise bad (LDL) cholesterol and increase the risk of athero-sclerotic coronary heart disease. Red meat also is high in omega-6 fatty acids. Whereas omega-3 fatty acids, found in cold-water fish, for example, help reduce inflammation in the body and have protective effects, omega-6 fatty acids do the opposite—they actually promote inflammation in the body. It is important to keep a healthy ratio of omega-3 to omega-6 fat in the diet, something that is woefully out of balance in the American diet.

> Research has shown that red meat consumption is linked to:
>
> - Cancer (colorectal, breast, prostate, and pancreatic)
> - Diabetes
> - Elevated cholesterol
> - Heart disease
> - Hypertension
> - Chronic Inflammation

One of the largest studies looking at the dangers of meat consumption on dying prematurely was reported several years ago.

The study of more than 500,000 middle-aged and elderly Americans found that those who consumed four ounces of red meat a day (the equivalent of about a small hamburger) were more than 30% more likely to die during the 10 years they were followed, mostly from heart disease and cancer. Red meat included beef, pork, and all processed meat.

The study's lead author, Dr. Rashmi Sinha of the National Cancer Institute, stated, "The bottom line is we found an association between red meat and processed meat and an increased risk of mortality."

In contrast, routine consumption of fish, chicken, turkey, and other poultry decreased the risk of death.

Barry M. Popkin, PhD, a professor of global nutrition at the University of North Carolina, wrote an editorial accompanying the study and stated, "This is a slam-dunk to say that, 'Yes, indeed, if people want to be healthy and live longer, consume less red and processed meat.'"

Why is the consumption of red meat so unhealthy? There are many explanations:

- Cooking red meat generates cancer-causing compounds; red meat is also high in saturated fat, which has been associated with atherosclerosis and cancer.
- Meat is high in heme iron, also believed to promote cancer and atherosclerotic cardiovascular disease.

- People who eat red meat are more likely to have high blood pressure and elevated cholesterol, which increases the risk of heart disease.
- Processed meats contain substances known as nitrosamines, which have been linked to cancer.

New research continues to prove this point. Research out of the Harvard School of Public Health's Department of Nutrition looked at what would happen when women started changing the proteins in their diet. They published in *Circulation: Journal of the American Heart Association* that women who had two servings of red meat per day had a 30% greater risk of developing heart disease compared to women who opted for one-half of a serving per day.

Moreover, women who substituted one serving of red meat per day for one serving of nuts lowered their risk of developing coronary heart disease by 30%! Substituting fish for red meat lowered the risk by 24%! This landmark study looked at these dietary behaviors in more than 84,000 women over a period of 26 years.

Additional studies shed light on the inherent dangers of following a typical Western or American diet. During World War II, there was a marked reduction in the incidence of heart attacks in Europe. Researchers have linked this finding to the marked reduction in red meat and dairy consumption during this time. When the war ended and red meat and dairy consumption returned, so did the heart attacks!

Research has also shown that following the toxic American diet leads to atherosclerotic coronary artery disease at a young age. The majority of the young soldiers (18 to 20 years old) killed in Vietnam and Korea already had established atherosclerotic plaques in their coronary arteries at the time of autopsy.

Caution: Trans Fat in Milk and Beef

A recent Norwegian study presented at the European Society of Cardiology's EuroPrevent meeting in Geneva Switzerland revealed that small amounts of naturally occurring (ruminant) trans fats in milk and beef boost cardiac risk more than expected. The study of more than 71,000 people followed for 25 years showed that men with the highest consumption of ruminant trans fats were 41% more likely to die from coronary heart disease, and women with the highest ruminant transfat intake were twice as likely to die from coronary heart disease.

Other Meat Dangers: Well-Done is No Good

The trouble with meat is that it's not just the saturated fats and omega-6 fats that are harming you. Depending on what *kinds* of meats you like to eat and how you cook them, you could be putting yourself at even greater risk.

Eating well-done meat has been found to increase the risk of certain cancers. Meats cooked at high temperatures generate chemicals called heterocyclic amines (HCAs). These HCAs are known to cause various cancers, including lung, bladder, colorectal, stomach, pancreatic, and others.

In one 12-year study from the prestigious University of Texas MD Anderson Cancer Center, individuals in the group who ate the most red meat were 1.5 times more likely to develop bladder cancer than those who ate the least red meat. Strikingly, the degree to which the meats were cooked also increased one's risk. Individuals who favored well-done meats were twice as likely to develop bladder cancer compared to meat-eaters who liked their cuts rare. Similar red-meat-eating patterns are also linked to lung cancer.

Other Meat Dangers: Processed is Problematic (and Prohibited)

To stay healthy, you must also avoid processed meats. What I mean by processed is any meat that has been altered from its natural state for the sake of preserving its shelf life. Many researchers define processed meat as being preserved by smoking, curing, or salting, or with the addition of chemical preservatives.

Processed meats include:

- Bacon
- Hot dogs
- Deli or luncheon meats
- Salami
- Sausage

Do you need more proof? Take a look at this study, possibly the largest of its kind ever done to date. In 2010, the Harvard School of Public Health analyzed 20 studies covering a total of more than 1.2 million people from 10 countries. Researchers found that eating just one serving of processed meat per day was associated with a 42% higher risk of heart disease and 19% higher risk of developing diabetes.

The researchers noted in their article, published in *Circulation*, that the processed meats had, on average, four times more sodium and 50% more nitrate preservatives than unprocessed meats.

Eastern Diets Compared

A landmark study conducted by scientist T. Colin Campbell was one of the first to shine the spotlight on how toxic the typical meat-laden Western diet is. He looked at mortality data from 50 diseases from more than 130 villages in rural mainland China.

What he and colleagues found was quite interesting. Compared to the U.S., the Chinese villagers consumed almost half the fat, only 10% of the meat, and three times more fiber than Americans. When looking at cardiovascular parameters, the mean cholesterol count for the Chinese villagers was 127 compared to 203 for the U.S. population aged 20–74. And death from coronary artery disease was almost 17 times greater for U.S. men and almost 6 times greater for U.S. women compared to the respective villagers.

Lastly, Dr. Stanley Hazen and his colleagues at the Cleveland Clinic have conducted research on red meat and cardiovascular disease. They concluded that red meat consumption leads to the production of TMAO (trimethylamine N-oxide) by the gut microbiome. TMAO then enters the bloodstream and increases the risk of atherosclerotic cardiovascular disease (heart attack and stroke) and vascular thrombosis (blood clots). Following a Mediterranean dietary pattern lowered TMAO levels.

Meat in Moderation

Based on my own experience and the overwhelming data showing the serious dangers of eating too much red meat, I recommend to my patients that if they are going to eat red meat, choose lean cuts, avoid cured or processed meats altogether (e.g., bacon, deli meat, hot dogs), and eat small portions (no bigger than a deck of playing cards) no more than once a week.

Therefore, if you want to protect your heart and your overall health, the key is avoiding frequent red-meat consumption. The traditional Mediterranean diet is associated with infrequent red meat consumption (once or twice a month), and those that follow this diet have a fraction of the heart disease (and cancer) compared to the typical Western (or American) diet.

> - Avoid regular red meat consumption (limit intake to four ounces two to four times a month)
> - Avoid processed meat
> - Consume fish (omega-3 rich) and poultry (skinless chicken or turkey) several times per week

Dairy

One of our most prevalent American myths is that drinking whole milk every day is good for you. Besides increasing cholesterol due to its cholesterol and saturated fat content, whole milk has been a big contributor to the obesity epidemic in America. Note that three 8-ounce glasses of whole milk contains 450 calories and 15 grams of saturated fat!

In addition, the hormones given to cows to increase their milk production, as well as the antibiotics they're fed to prevent infection, have also been found in blood samples of milk drinkers.

Regular milk consumption may increase the risk of:

- Diabetes
- GI disturbances (due to lactose intolerance)
- Heart disease
- Multiple sclerosis
- Ovarian cancer
- Prostate cancer

If you consume cow's milk, switch from whole milk to skim milk (in moderation). Likewise, choose low-fat or fat-free cheese and yogurt.

Many milk alternatives are now available, including soy milk and almond milk. Because soy milk contains phytoestrogens, recent research has cautioned that it may not be suitable for consumption by women with a family history of breast cancer.

I recommend almond milk. Almonds are rich in nutrients, and almond milk has no cholesterol, saturated fat, or trans fat. Not to mention, almond milk is great for those who are lactose intolerant. Best of all, almond milk is low caloric and delicious!

Whey: A Wonderful Alternative Protein

If you want to include non-meat sources of protein in your diet, whey protein is an excellent option. Whey protein is the collection of proteins from milk when cheese is made. But what makes whey protein so good is that it is a complete protein, meaning it contains all nine essential amino acids. Essential amino acids cannot be made by the body, so we must get enough through our diet to support protein synthesis. Whey protein is highly bioavailable, meaning it is easy for your body to digest and assimilate into the needed ingredients.

Research also shows that whey can help manage blood glucose levels. When whey protein was given in combination with a pure glucose drink, blood glucose levels were significantly lowered compared to when just the glucose drink was consumed. And all lean proteins have a thermogenic effect, increasing the basal metabolic rate (the amount of energy your body burns at rest).

The Mediterranean Diet: The Optimal Diet for Heart Health

In contrast to the toxic American Diet, the Mediterranean diet is very low in saturated fat and contains no trans fat. It consists of fruits, vegetables, olive oil, whole grains, legumes, nuts, fish, poultry, and red wine (in moderation) with food. Red meat is eaten infrequently, and sugar, refined starches, and processed foods are avoided. The result is that those who naturally enjoy this type of diet have a reduced risk of heart disease. In addition, this diet lowers the risk of metabolic syndrome, diabetes, hypertension, Alzheimer's disease, cancer, and a number of other diseases.

So what is the Mediterranean diet, and how is it so different than our American or Western diet? All of the foods found in a traditional Mediterranean diet are non-processed and can be found in any grocery store. There is nothing exotic about them. In sum, the Mediterranean diet is plentiful in vitamins, fiber, and antioxidants required for good health. It includes many foods that have now been shown to reduce inflammation, whereas the typical American diet *promotes* inflammation. Decreasing inflammation lowers the risk of heart disease, cancer, diabetes, and a host of other diseases that are linked to chronic low-grade inflammation.

Mediterranean Diet Pyramid

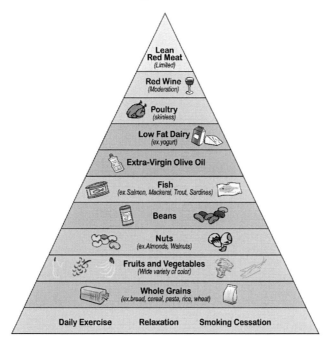

Foods typical of a traditional Mediterranean diet:

- Nuts, beans, and whole grains
- Vegetables (wide variety)
- Fresh fruit
- Cold-water fish
- Olive oil
- Red wine with dinner

The Mediterranean diet and lifestyle also provides a great foundation for healthy living that promotes weight loss and maintenance. For these reasons, I have recommended this healthy diet and lifestyle for my patients for more than thirty years.

Weight Loss and the Mediterranean Diet

A Mediterranean diet can be a great tool for weight loss. People who live in the Mediterranean region and follow a traditional Mediterranean diet and lifestyle are much leaner than their American counterparts who consume a typical Western diet.

This diet plan and the wonderful food it offers promotes weight loss in a number of ways:

- High fiber: the consumption of food with a high-fiber content (like fruits, vegetables, beans, nuts, and whole grains) leads to feelings of satiety, or being full and satisfied.

- Omega-3 thermogenesis: the consumption of omega-3 fats has also been shown to help achieve weight loss through a process known as thermogenesis, or heat release, following the metabolism of fat.
- Less sugar: The Mediterranean diet contains complex instead of simple carbohydrates, and refined sugar is avoided. A traditional Mediterranean diet contains no significant refined sugar. That compares to 25% of our diets today.

The Skinny on Sweeteners

Until recently, options for calorie-free sweeteners had all been chemical. Equal, Sweet'N Low, and Splenda are all chemical derivatives of sugar, but are not natural.

The good news is that zero-calorie sweeteners are now being made from the stevia plant and are completely natural. Leaves from the stevia plant, from which the sweeteners are made, are known to be 30 times sweeter than table sugar. Stevia can now be found at most major grocery stores. A little goes a long way, so try some in your tea or coffee. And you can even use it in baking.

Building Your New Diet: A Mediterranean Mix

Let's now take a look at the healthy and delicious foods of the Mediterranean diet.

Good Fats: Omega-3 Fatty Acids

Omega-3 fat is an important component of the Mediterranean diet because it is something the average American doesn't consume enough of. It has been suggested that up to 90% of Americans are deficient in omega-3 fatty acids.

Why should this matter? Whereas omega-3 fat (found in walnuts, flaxseed oil, and fish) is anti-in-flammatory, omega-6 fat (found in vegetable oil and much of today's red meat) is pro-inflammatory. The omega-6/omega-3 ratio should be two to one; how-ever, due to the decrease in omega-3 intake and the increase in omega-6 intake, that ratio for many men and women is somewhere between 10:1 and 20:1!

This drastic imbalance in the ratio of omega-3 to omega-6 fats is strongly linked to an increase in:

- Acne
- Allergies
- Arthritis
- Asthma
- Cancer
- Depression
- Diabetes
- Heart rhythm disorders
- Heart disease
- Hypertension
- Inflammatory bowel disease
- Sudden cardiac death

The Mediterranean diet naturally resets this ratio to healthy levels by providing your body with ample amounts of omega-3 fat.

Olive Oil

Olive oil is the "soul" of the Mediterranean diet and provides the taste and flavor of Mediterranean dishes. It is made by crushing and then pressing olives. Olive oil is rich in monounsaturated fat and is used in place of butter or margarine.

Olive oil also has a favorable impact on our cholesterol. Besides decreasing our total cholesterol, it also lowers the bad (LDL) cholesterol and makes it less susceptible to oxidative damage by free radicals. The good (HDL) cholesterol is maintained or increased with olive oil consumption, and the total cholesterol to HDL ratio is improved. Olive oil has also been shown to have beneficial anti-inflammatory, antioxidant, and anti-thrombotic properties.

A Mediterranean diet with olive oil also helps with weight loss. A study in Boston revealed that a diet which included olive oil and nuts resulted in sustained weight loss over 18 months compared to a low-fat diet. People also stayed on the diet longer because they did not feel deprived.

A recent study by the Harvard School of Public Health published in the April 2020 *Journal of the American College of Cardiology* found that higher olive-oil intake was associated with lower risk of cardiovascular disease in two large prospective cohorts of U.S. men and women. The substitution of margarine, butter, mayonnaise, and dairy fat with olive oil leads to a lower risk of coronary heart disease and cardiovascular disease.

One word of caution: olive oil is high caloric (100 calories per tablespoon), so use in moderation—drizzle, don't pour!

Vinegar

Vinegar has long been a staple in the Mediterranean diet. It is frequently used with olive oil, and for a good reason. Vinegar leads to satiety. In addition, vinegar helps manage blood sugar and insulin levels. Vinegar helps to reduce blood glucose by delaying gastric emptying, which slows the absorption of carbohydrates.

Researchers found that when vinegar was served with white bread, blood sugar and insulin levels were lower compared to white bread consumed without vinegar. In addition, vinegar increased satiety. These findings were published in the *European Journal of Clinical Nutrition*.

Fresh Fruits and Vegetables

Go to any supermarket in the Mediterranean basin and you will find a bountiful supply of fresh, native fruits and vegetables. Fruits and vegetables contain an abundance of vitamins, minerals, fiber, and complex carbohydrates that lower the risk of heart disease and cancer. They also contain phytonutrients, concentrated in the skins, which help fight disease and improve health.

Some of my favorite heart-healthy fruits and vegetables:

- Artichoke
- Zucchini
- Eggplant
- Spinach
- Red Peppers

- Mushrooms
- Garlic
- Olives
- Chickpeas
- Orange

- Apples
- Grapes
- Pomegranate

In a large European study involving 313,074 men and women from eight European countries who were followed for more than eight years, those who ate at least eight portions of fruits and vegetables per day had a 22% lower risk of dying from coronary heart disease compared to those who ate fewer than three portions a day. Interestingly, just adding one additional fruit or vegetable portion per day decreased risk by 4%. The results of this study were published in the *European Heart Journal*.

Whole Grains

Whole grains are unrefined and have not gone through many rounds of processing and hence have more fiber, nutrients, and a heartier, nuttier texture. A whole grain kernel consists of an outer layer, the bran (fiber); a middle layer (complex carbohydrates and protein); and an inner layer (vitamins, minerals, and proteins). The process of refining destroys the outer and inner layer of the grain, resulting in a stripped version that is devoid of the healthy fiber and protective vitamins and phytochemicals. Because of this, whole grains rather than refined grains have been shown to decrease the risk of heart disease and diabetes.

A recent study conducted by Harvard's School of Public Health found that eating five or more servings of white rice per week is associated with an increased risk of type 2 diabetes. But if the white rice is changed to brown rice and eaten just two or more times per week, the risk is lowered. When the white rice was replaced with other whole grains, such as whole wheat and barley, the risk decreased even more.

Excellent Sources of Whole Grains:

- Wheat
- Oats
- Brown Rice
- Quinoa

- Rye
- Amaranth
- Spelt
- Millet

Health Benefits of Nuts and Beans

Nuts are an excellent source of good fats and protein. Almonds are rich in fiber and walnuts contain heart-healthy omega-3 fat. Several clinical trials have demonstrated that consuming nuts in moderation on a regular basis leads to lower cholesterol, a decreased risk of coronary heart disease, and a significant reduction in the risk of heart attack. I recommend a handful of natural raw almonds every day as a satisfying and nutritious midday snack.

Beans and other legumes are another good source of protein and fiber. They, too, have been shown to lower the risk of heart disease, cancer, and diabetes when consumed regularly.

Fish

What would a Mediterranean diet be without fish? The Mediterranean Sea offers a variety of omega-3 rich seafood that is exceptionally healthy. When looking for the optimal health benefits, the oily, cold-water fish are the best, as they have high levels of omega-3 fat. In particular, salmon is an excellent choice, as well as albacore tuna, herring, sardines, shad, trout, flounder (or sole), and pollock.

A note of caution, however: avoid eating swordfish, tilefish, shark, and mackerel, as these tend to have very high mercury levels. It is particularly important that pregnant and nursing women and young children avoid fish with high mercury levels. Always discuss nutritional recommendations, including fish consumption, with your health-care provider.

The omega-3 and mercury content of popular fish and shellfish consumed in the United States

	Mean mercury level in parts per million (ppm)	Omega-3 fatty acids (grams per 3-oz. serving)
Canned tuna (light)	0.12	0.17–0.24
Shrimp	ND*	0.29
Pollock	0.06	0.45
Salmon (fresh, frozen)	0.01	1.1–1.9
Cod	0.11	0.15–0.24
Catfish	0.05	0.22–0.3
Clams	ND*	0.25
Flounder or sole	0.05	0.48
Crabs	0.06	0.27–0.40
Scallops	0.05	0.18–0.34

Other common seafoods

	Mean mercury level in parts per million (ppm)	Omega-3 fatty acids (grams per 3-oz. serving)
Lobster	0.31	0.07–0.46
Grouper	0.55	0.23

Fish with the highest levels of mercury (about 1 ppm Hg)

	Mean mercury level in parts per million (ppm)	Omega-3 fatty acids (grams per 3-oz. serving)
Shark	0.99	0.83
Swordfish	0.97	0.97
Tilefish (golden bass or golden snapper)	1.45	0.90
King mackerel	0.73	0.36

Alcohol–The Double-Edged Sword

Up to this point, I've covered red meat, dairy, fruits and vegetables, fish, olive oil and vinegar, and more. So now I offer up a toast to the good life with a glass of red wine. Cultures with the longest longevity— such as those living in the Mediterranean, Okinawa, Sardinia, Andorra—all have been known to drink small amounts of alcohol with their afternoon or evening meal.

Countless studies have shown the cardiovascular benefits of drinking a glass of red wine with dinner. One reason may be that red wine raises HDL (good) cholesterol, decreases clotting, lowers inflammation, and reduces oxidation of LDL (bad) cholesterol. In addition, red wine also contains resveratrol, a powerful antioxidant.

But remember, alcohol, including red wine, only has cardiovascular benefits when consumed in moderation—one glass per day for a woman and two glasses per day for a man (serving size: 5 ounces of wine; 12 ounces of beer; 1.5 ounces of spirits).

What is most interesting is new data showing that other types of alcohol, including beer and spirits, also provide protection against heart disease. In the large INTER-HEART study involving 27,000 people from 52 countries, light to moderate drinking reduced the incidence of heart attack in men and women in all age groups. Moderate alcohol consumption also decreases the risk of ischemic stroke and type 2 diabetes.

An evening drink has also been shown to be beneficial in those with cardiovascular risk factors, such as hypertension. In one study that tracked 11,711 men with hypertension over 16 years, one drink per day reduced the risk of a heart attack by about 30%. To drive home the point about moderation, though, those who had more than two drinks daily showed increases in blood pressure.

Therefore, alcohol consumed in moderation lowers cardiovascular risk; however, men and women who exceed moderation raise their risk of cardiovascular disease—as well as other diseases, including liver disease and cancer.

A recent study demonstrated that even small amounts of alcohol can increase the risk of atrial fibrillation, a heart rhythm disorder that can lead to heart failure and stroke. As a preventive cardiologist, I do not encourage my patients who don't drink alcohol to start drinking in order to reduce their risk of a heart attack—there are better ways to lower risk without the potential adverse effects of alcohol. I do, however, advise my patients who already consume alcohol to do so in moderation.

- Don't start drinking alcohol to prevent disease.
- If you do drink alcohol, do so in moderation, and discuss the pros and cons of drinking with your personal physician.
- Moderation is no more than one drink for a woman or two drinks for a man in a 24-hour period.
- One drink is 12 ounces of beer; 5 ounces of wine; 1.5 ounces of spirits.

The Dark Side of Alcohol Consumption

- Auto accidents and other accidents
- Addiction
- Increase risk of cancer
- Cirrhosis of the liver
- Heart rhythm disturbances
- Depression
- Insomnia
- Memory Loss

Have a "Spot of Tea"–your heart will thank you!

Don't let your love affair with coffee blind you to the benefits of tea. Tea as a beverage dates back to about 2737 BC in China. All teas come from the *camellia sinensis* plant, and the processing of the leaves is what determines its type and color. Both coffee and tea contain antioxidants and chemicals that have been found to reduce the risk of diabetes, gallstones, and kidney stones. But it is tea that contains substances that help reduce the risk of heart disease and cancer.

One question I am often asked is whether the kind of tea matters. The answer is yes. Green tea has been lauded as the healthiest because it is made from young tea leaves that are immediately steamed, rolled, and dried, providing more antioxidant power and boosting its health benefits. Black tea comes from leaves that are exposed to oxygen for two to four hours. White tea is the least processed and lowest in caffeine. But research has shown that black tea, rooibos, and white tea also protect against cancer and heart disease.

In fact, researchers at the University of California in Los Angeles conducted a meta-analysis of several studies comparing stroke protection in green tea and black tea drinkers. The results suggested that daily consumption of either green or black tea equaling three cups per day could help prevent the onset of ischemic stroke.

A very recent analysis by Chinese researchers of 18 tea studies published in the *American Journal of Clinical Nutrition* determined that while black tea is healthy, green tea is best if you want to decrease your risk of dying from heart disease. In the analysis, an increase of green tea consumption of one cup per day was associated with a 10% decrease in the risk of developing coronary artery disease!

To release tea's strongest health benefits, brew it yourself, using either the leaves or a tea bag, and let it steep in the cup for three to five minutes. Keep in mind that while herbal teas may be more flavorful, pure tea packs a stronger antioxidant punch.

Cinnamon

When I say cinnamon, if you're thinking holidays, apple cider, and pumpkin pie, think again. Cinnamon is a great spice that not only flavors all kinds of foods (check many Chinese and Indian recipes!) but also has some impressive health benefits.

Ground cinnamon is made from the bark of the cinnamon tree, and it contains three types of essential oils that provide it with health-boosting properties, as well as a wide range of other active substances. These oils act as an anticoagulant, preventing blood from forming dangerous clots; they have anti-inflammatory properties; and they enhance the ability of diabetics to metabolize sugar.

In fact, less than a half-teaspoon a day of cinnamon can lower glucose levels and improve cholesterol balance in people at high risk for diabetes and coronary heart disease.

Specific Health Benefits of a Traditional Mediterranean Diet

This chapter is about building a new dietary and nutritional foundation for you to lose weight, or maintain the weight you are at, while reaping the wealth of health benefits a Mediterranean-style diet has to offer, including protection against diseases other than heart disease and cancer.

The Mediterranean Diet helps prevent:

- Cardiovascular disease
- Hypertension
- Diabetes
- Cancer
- Alzheimer's disease
- Allergies
- Asthma
- Metabolic syndrome
- Inflammatory bowel disease
- Depression and anxiety
- Autoimmune diseases
- Neurodegenerative diseases

In fact, researchers from Italy recently looked at all studies through June 2010 that assessed the benefits of the Mediterranean diet and published them in the *American Journal of Clinical Nutrition.* They found that the Mediterranean diet was associated with a statistically significant reduction of overall mortality, as well as cardiovascular mortality, cancer mortality, and neurodegenerative diseases.

Because of this, I wanted to call attention to some of the specific studies that highlight the power of this age-old way of enjoying food:

Cardiovascular Health

We've already mentioned some of the cardio-protective effects of the Mediterranean diet. Early landmark studies confirming the benefits include:

The Lyon Diet Heart Study

This study compared a Mediterranean diet to a control diet resembling the American Heart Association's recommendations for heart attack survivors. The control diet is still considered by many to be healthy since it restricted total fat to no more than 30% of total calories, saturated fat to no more than 10% of total calories, and cholesterol to less than 300 mg/day. The Mediterranean diet, however, was healthier. It had:

- More whole grain bread, more vegetables, and more fish

- less beef, lamb, and pork (replaced with poultry)
- no day without fruit
- butter and cream were replaced with margarine high in alpha-linolenic acid (an omega-3 fat)

The Mediterranean diet proved to be far superior—it was associated with a 70% decrease in the risk of death and a 73% decrease in risk of recurrent cardiac events, such as heart attack or sudden cardiac death, compared to the control diet plan.

The Singh Indo-Mediterranean Diet Study

This study placed 499 patients at risk for coronary heart disease on an Indo-Mediterranean diet. Results showed that the diet change reduced serum cholesterol and also significantly reduced heart attacks and sudden cardiac death. Subjects also had fewer cardiovascular events than those on a conventional diet.

The NIH-AARP Diet and Health Study

This large study looked at more than 350,000 men and women in the United States to evaluate the impact of a Mediterranean diet on their health. The findings, published in 2007 Archives of Internal Medicine, demonstrated that a Mediterranean diet not only lowered the risk of heart attacks, but it also significantly reduced the death rate from a variety of diseases, including cardiovascular disease and cancer.

These results provide strong evidence for a beneficial effect of higher conformity with the Mediterranean dietary pattern on the risk of death from all causes.

Protective Against Cancers

The beauty of the traditional Mediterranean diet is that it is synergistic in how it protects the body. This means that each component is not only nutritious in and of itself, but when they are combined with one another, they act together to become even more effective. They are more powerful in combination than if they were eaten separately. This may help explain why this diet has shown protection against certain types of cancers.

Recent research from Harvard University is proving this is still the case in Greece. In 14,800 Greek women who were followed for ten years, those who followed their region's traditional diet most closely were 22% less likely to develop breast cancer than those who ate less traditional diets. The results were published in the *American Journal of Clinical Nutrition* and were found to apply to a subset of the women who were past menopause. The data add to other research showing protection against colon, stomach, and prostate cancer.

Protective against Alzheimer's Disease

Dr. Nikolaos Scarmeas and colleagues from Columbia University Medical Center in New York demonstrated in 2006 that a Mediterranean diet reduced the risk of developing Alzheimer's disease by 68%. Recent updates to this study confirm the original results and also show that it may reduce the risk of mild cognitive impairment.

A third, related study by Scarmeas looking at diet, exercise, and Alzheimer's risk in elderly French participants showed that the greater the adherence to a Mediterranean diet or the more physical activity the participants engaged in, the lower the risk for developing Alzheimer's disease.

Reduced Depression Rates

The benefits of the Mediterranean diet go beyond reduced rates of heart disease, helping prevent cancer and offering protection against Alzheimer's disease. Interestingly, lifetime incidences of depression in the Mediterranean countries also have been found to be lower than in Northern European countries, according to research published in *Archives of General Psychiatry* by Spanish scientists looking at rates of depression. In approximately 10,000 healthy Spanish people followed for six years, those who adhered to a Mediterranean diet had a 30% reduction in the risk of becoming depressed compared to those who did not follow a Mediterranean-style diet.

Not All Foods Are Created Equal

Unfortunately, many of the foods that make up our traditional Western diet are toxic to our bodies. Consuming unhealthy food is like putting diesel fuel in a gasoline powered car—it simply does not work. We are not genetically programmed to function on processed food!

In fact, processed food is directly related to the ever-increasing spikes in obesity, hypertension, diabetes, heart disease, stroke, and yes, death. The toxic American diet is loaded with preservatives, sodium, refined sugar, and bad fats. So what's the alternative? Become Mediterranean!

Research study after research study has shown that those following a traditional Mediterranean diet and lifestyle suffer significantly less heart disease and are far less likely to die from a heart attack. In fact, one of the oldest studies showed that Greek men living on the island of Crete were 90% less likely to die from a heart attack than their American counterparts.

But even more compelling is research showing that those who switch to a Mediterranean diet and lifestyle share in the same health benefits (including fewer heart attacks, a longer life expectancy, and a reduced risk of cancer), regardless of where they live or what their diets were like before. Why?

We know that there are certain foods, and food components, that can change your cardiovascular disease risk.

There are literally dozens of "super foods" in the Mediterranean diet that are absolute musts to start eating—not only because they are great for you, but because they taste good too!

A Few Mediterranean Musts!

Try these heart-healthy foods instead of their Toxic Trade-offs

Breakfast: Oatmeal instead of sugary cereal

Snack: A handful of almonds instead of potato chips

Sweet: A platter of fresh fruit

Alcohol: Red wine in moderation

Meat: Grilled salmon instead of grilled steak

Spreads/Oil: Virgin olive oil and vinegar instead of butter or margarine

---

So take note of what you're eating, and stock up on these Mediterranean favorites.

A selected menu plan and recipes from *The Complete Mediterranean Diet* are listed in the supplement section of the book.

Key Points

> The "toxic" American diet is highly processed, calorie dense, and nutrient depleted.

- The Mediterranean diet was selected as the best overall dietary eating pattern in America by US News and World Report.

- The Mediterranean diet has been shown in clinical trials to lower the risk of heart attack and stroke, lower the risk of Alzheimer's disease, lower blood pressure, lower inflammation, lower LDL cholesterol and atherogenic particles, improve HDL cholesterol function, reduce plaque formation in the arteries, lower the risk of plaque rupture, lower the risk of sudden cardiac death, lower cancer risk, improve longevity, and help achieve and maintain optimal body weight.

- Omega-3 fatty acids from omega-3-rich fish (e.g., salmon, sardines, tuna, trout) have been shown to lower cardiovascular risk and prevent sudden cardiac death.

- Extra virgin olive oil to replace butter and margarine has been shown to lower the risk of coronary heart disease.

- Avoid alcohol consumption—if you do drink, do so in moderation (e.g., 5 oz red wine with main meal of the day).

- The Mediterranean diet reduces blood sugar and lowers the risk of insulin resistance and diabetes

➢ Consume a wide variety of fruits and vegetables

➢ Avoid processed carbohydrates, including refined starches and sugar

➢ Consume red meat in moderation; avoid processed meat

➢ Consume whole grains; avoid processed grains

➢ Consume fiber (e.g., beans, legumes, seeds, nuts)—at least 25 grams/day for women and 35 grams/day for men

➢ Main beverage throughout the day is water

CHAPTER 7

Physical Activity for a Healthy Heart

How familiar is this scenario? You're at the other end of the house, and the phone starts ringing. You sprint to pick it up in time, answering with a "Hello" that leaves you needing a few moments to catch your breath and hoping that the person on the other end can't tell that you are panting.

In the 30 seconds it probably took you to move from your present task to pick up the phone, your heart and body performed several functions. Your brain told your muscles you needed to move, and quickly. Your lungs started expanding to increase the rate of oxygen you consumed, and your respiratory rate increased. And your heart went into overdrive to supply extra blood and oxygen to the muscles to get them moving so you could answer the phone in time.

While sprinting to answer the phone can't be considered exercise, in some ways, it is a mini-fitness test. Fitness has long been defined as the ability to perform daily tasks without fatigue or undue distress. But technological advances and a culture of efficiency have literally moved us from a life of daily functional activity to being almost immobile on the office chair or couch. And for all the strides we've made in the name of technological progress, we have taken two steps backward due to our poor nutrition and sedentary lifestyle.

Exercise is Essential

It's not that the technological advancements of our modern lives are bad. Certainly, we've improved our quality of life, become a global society, and from a medical standpoint, have developed amazing tools to save lives. But today, we spend so much of our lives sitting—sitting at work toiling away at our computers, sitting at home in front of the television, sitting in our cars as we motor from place to place. It's hardly an idea of fitness.

And when viewed from an anatomical and physiological perspective, this inactivity is absolutely contrary to what the body was designed for. The body is designed to move—stretch, flex, bend, twist, jump, run, and more! Movement promotes circulation of blood to all of the organs, improved oxygen capacity, increased body heat and detoxification through sweating and other filtration methods. It's no wonder that all of this physical inactivity is directly linked to poor health outcomes, specifically obesity, diabetes, heart attack, stroke, cancer and more.

Truthfully, we've known how detrimental inactivity is for some time. Going all the way back to

1953, a British physician by the name of Jeremy Morris and colleagues studied conductors working on London's double-decker buses who climbed nearly 600 stairs per workday. Morris compared them to bus drivers, who sat driving a bus for 90% of the day, and found that the conductors had half as many heart attacks as the bus drivers.

Yet, we live even more sedentary lives today than we did almost 60 years ago when Jeremy Morris did his research! What does this mean? It means that today we must make a conscious choice to be physically active if we want to live long, healthy lives.

Chances are, if you have opened this book, you already have decided to choose a healthier lifestyle, and hopefully that includes looking forward to regular exercise.

Instead of sitting on the couch and watching television, each and every night, get up and walk in place for 30 minutes while watching your favorite show. Get moving!

The "Heart" Truth

The truth is, exercise is essential for heart health. There are no shortcuts, and to try to look for any would be depriving your mind, your body, and your heart of amazing benefits!

That's because exercise really works. And not just for the young, for the fit, or for the accomplished. Study after study has shown that your body reaps the benefits of exercise, even after one session! It's so effective that the Institute of Medicine has recommended that physicians start prescribing exercise instead of, or in combination with, certain medications for a variety of conditions. Sound crazy? It's not.

Take a recent study in a high-risk group: Elderly patients ages 65–83 with controlled type 2 diabetes, high blood pressure, and high blood cholesterol. Definitely a high-risk population. A geriatric specialist at the University of British Columbia, Dr. Kenneth Madden, decided to see if three months of exercise could improve the stiffness and elasticity of participants' arteries. Increased arterial stiffness is associated with adverse cardiac events like heart attack and stroke. Participants either did nothing and remained sedentary or exercised for one hour three times a week on treadmills or cycling machines with supervision. After the three months, the exercisers had a 20% reduction in arterial stiffness. That was a clinically meaningful reduction that most cardiologists would agree offers protection against future heart attacks.

Exercise and Hypertension

While we're talking about our arteries and how exercise and regular movement can keep them flexible, let's talk about blood pressure. Your blood pressure is the measure of the force of the blood against the artery wall as it moves through your body. When you have your blood pressure taken, you are given two numbers, read as one number over the other. The top number is your systolic pressure, and it measures the pressure of the blood against the artery wall when your heart contracts, and the bottom number is the diastolic pressure, which measures the pressure when the heart relaxes between beats. A normal blood pressure is 120/80 mmHg or lower. If your blood pressure is chronically higher than 130/80 mmHg, then you have a condition called stage one hypertension, and greater than 140/90 is stage two hypertension. Hypertension is extremely common today. Most of us know someone with hypertension; in fact, more than 50 million Americans deal with it on a daily basis. Yet we don't have to. It is usually preventable.

Hypertension can lead to:

- Heart attack
- Stroke
- Kidney failure
- Aortic aneurysm

Patient Story: Beth

Beth was referred to my office by her primary care physician for evaluation and treatment of her elevated cholesterol, blood sugar, and blood pressure. As a

49-year-old legal secretary and mother of two teenage boys, she was now taking prescription medications on a daily basis for the first time in her life. She was familiar with risk factors for heart disease, as her husband had a heart attack several years ago.

Needless to say, Beth was not happy about her elevated risk of heart attack, stroke, and diabetes, nor was she happy about the expense and side effects of blood pressure and cholesterol medications. She told me that her body weight was normal for most of her life; however, she'd gained 25 pounds over the past several years, and she was now overweight. Most interesting, she stated that she had always been active and exercised on a regular basis. Her favorite activities were walking in the park with friends, swimming, and bike riding. Unfortunately, due to her hectic schedule, she no longer engaged in regular exercise and found herself watching TV and movies most evenings and on the weekend.

I encouraged Beth to begin a Mediterranean diet and reduce her intake of refined sugar, saturated fat, and salt. In addition, I advised her to begin a walking program of 30 to 45 minutes a day. She purchased a pedometer and walked at least 10,000 steps a day.

Last but not least, she performed meditation in the form of the "relaxation response" for 15 minutes, twice a day. Six weeks after Beth began her exercise, diet, and stress management recommendations, her blood pressure, cholesterol, and blood sugar levels improved, and I began weaning her off her medications.

Four months later, Beth was completely off prescription medications, and her laboratory values and blood pressure were normal. Best of all, Beth lost 26 pounds and reported more energy during the day and improved sleep at night. During her last visit, she told me that her life had been in a downward spiral, but it had now returned to normal. In fact, Beth told me that she regained something she had lost–a zest for life!

Dozens of clinical studies support the beneficial impact that exercise has on health. Regarding hypertension, the scientific literature shows that on average, exercise decreases blood pressure in about 75% of all people with hypertension. Clinical studies have demonstrated that those who engage in regular exercise significantly reduce their risk of a heart attack.

Cardiovascular Benefits of Regular Exercise:

- Lowers body weight
- Improves lipid profile: lowers triglycerides and LDL cholesterol and raises HDL cholesterol
- Lowers inflammation
- Lowers risk of blood clots
- Lowers stress hormones (adrenalin)
- Lowers blood pressure and heart rate
- Dilates the coronary arteries
- Improves collateral circulation

Exercise and Heart Attack

Like the early research of the London bus drivers, data proving that regular exercise can prevent heart attacks go back decades. Further proof came from a pivotal 1980 study of nearly 20,000 male Civil Service workers. Simply put, half as many men who engaged in exercise in their leisure time suffered heart attacks or died from a heart attack over an eight-year period compared to men who had little leisure time activity. Remarkably, the protective effect of exercise persisted even when the researchers accounted for smoking, obesity, family history of coronary heart disease, and existing hypertension. To quote the 1980 study abstract published in *The Lancet:*

> Men who engaged in vigorous sports, keep-fit, and the like during an initial survey in 1968–70 had an incidence of coronary heart disease in the next eight years somewhat less than half that of their colleagues who recorded no vigorous exercise. The generality of the advantage suggests that vigorous exercise is a natural defense of the body, with a protective effect on the aging heart against ischemia and its consequences.

In an article published in Circulation, researchers from Harvard released data from the 10-year

Women's Health Study that showed moderate exercise reduced the risk of heart disease by as much as 41%.

Exercise is so powerful, it even helps those with existing heart disease, including those who have already had a heart attack. If you have survived a heart attack, there is strong evidence to show that if you start exercising now, you can greatly improve your chances of preventing future heart attacks, as well as surviving a second one should it happen.

It is important to discuss exercise with your personal physician. If you have risk factors for heart disease, your doctor may want you to perform an exercise stress test prior to starting exercise or increased physical activity.

Exercise and Stroke

A stroke is an extremely debilitating cardiovascular event. It is the result of any interruption of blood to the brain, typically from a blocked or ruptured blood vessel that carries oxygen and nutrients to the brain. Stroke is the third-leading cause of death and the most common form of debilitating handicap for adults. Someone has a stroke about every 45 seconds, with women suffering strokes more often than men, according to the National Stroke Association.

Like a heart attack, a "brain attack" also has similar risk factors, including smoking, high blood pressure, and diabetes. Recovering from a stroke takes months and even years of rehabilitation, often without a full recovery.

As physicians, we like to think we know what is best for our patients. I know how important it is to eat well, exercise, and manage stress, particularly to mitigate a heart attack or stroke. Highlighting this, a large study done by Harvard researchers looked at whether exercise protected male physicians against a stroke. In the study, renowned epidemiologist and physician Dr. Charles Hennekens and colleagues followed more than 20,000 physicians for almost 12 years. Dr. Hennekens found that exercise vigorous enough to work up a sweat, even just once per week, decreased the risk of a stroke by 26% compared to the least active men.

Move it or Lose it

The good news is that because our bodies are designed to move, it's pretty easy be active! Most of us probably don't know that our bodies have over 600 skeletal muscles at our disposal. These skeletal muscles are what we use to do everything from blink and eat to sit, stand, run, and swim.

But these muscles serve another important function. Together, when they are activated in larger groups, they stimulate blood circulation throughout the body, helping to remove toxins as well as improve the efficiency of our lungs and heart.

Fit or Fat?

Clinical studies have shown that your physical activity level is a better predictor of a heart attack or adverse cardiac event than your body weight.

Take professional football players. They have muscle and many also have excess fat. So how healthy are they? Are they protected from heart disease and attacks?

Researchers at the University of Texas Southwestern Medical Center put those questions to the test with former players of the National Football League. What the researchers found was that all that fitness, regardless of the player's body fat, had paid off. They were better protected against heart disease compared to sedentary men their age despite the fact that most NFL players have a body mass index (BMI) that categorizes them as overweight or obese. The findings, which were published in the *American Journal of Cardiology*, showed that the retired NFL players had a significantly lower prevalence of diabetes, hypertension, and metabolic syndrome compared to their non-athletic peers.

So what this means is that it's more important to be fit and active and perhaps a bit overweight than thin and unfit. This does not mean that we should not strive to achieve ideal body weight. It does, however, stress the importance of achieving fitness as well as normal body weight for optimum health.

It is important to note that we don't have to run marathons to be fit. What is most important is that you do regular exercise consistently. For instance, walking briskly 30 to 45 minutes per day will lead to a level of fitness that reduces cardiovascular risk.

What is Visceral Fat?

Research also shows that exercise helps keep off the fat that we can't see, fat that resides in the abdominal cavity and around internal organs, which is otherwise known as *visceral fat* and is associated with many health risks. Exercise physiologists at the University of Alabama at Birmingham (UAB) found that as little as 80 minutes a week of aerobic or resistance training not only prevented weight gain but also inhibited a regain of harmful visceral (belly) fat one year after weight loss.

In the study, which was published in the journal *Obesity*, UAB exercise physiologist Gary Hunter, PhD, and his team randomly assigned 45 European-American and 52 African American women to three groups: aerobic training, resistance training, or no exercise, but all had a restricted diet. After losing weight, the researchers recorded participants total fat, abdominal subcutaneous fat, and visceral fat. Then participants in the two exercise groups were asked to continue exercising 40 minutes twice a week for one year. What the researchers found was that participants who continued exercising, despite slight overall weight gains, regained zero percent of the visceral fat, compared to a 33% regain of visceral fat for those who stopped exercising or didn't exercise at all.

What's important to note here is the large benefit gained from just two exercise sessions per week, a relatively small commitment.

Without a doubt, exercise and establishing a level of fitness is essential to protecting your heart and health. I have seen it time and time again with my own patients—once an exercise routine is started, warning signslike elevated blood sugar, high blood pressure, and high triglyceride and cholesterol levels drop, and the risk of heart attack is reduced. And research has proven it, too, in clinical studies worldwide.

Researchers have also been able to establish a relationship between how much exercise you do, measured in calories burned per week, and the degree of health benefit or protection one can achieve, specific to cardiovascular disease and death. Even patients who have already suffered a heart attack and started exercising survive longer than their non-exercising counterparts. Expending between 700 and 2000 extra calories a week through exercising provides the greatest protective effect, especially in those who mainly have been sedentary.

> ## Exercise is Medicine
>
> In 2007, the American Medical Association and the American College of Sports Medicine (ACSM) launched the "Exercise is Medicine" program to advocate and encourage doctors to prescribe exercise to their patients as treatment. According to a recent ACSM survey, nearly two-thirds of patients said they would be more interested in exercising to stay healthy if advised by their doctor.

Boost Your Endorphins!

Beyond restoring health to the heart, achieving longevity, and improving the quality of life, there are additional perks to staying physically active.

I'm sure you've heard of a runner's high? Joggers, runners, and walkers often refer to this phenomenon, which includes a state of euphoria when exercising. Aerobic activity, especially more cardiovascular endurance-based exercise, produces a release of endorphins in the body and brain, leaving you feeling happy!

Exercise also boosts your mood and helps beat depression the same way. And it has been shown to be an effective prescription to treat anxiety, with similar if not better results when compared to traditional medicinal therapy.

Regular exercise also helps those who want to quit smoking. Exercise can help, especially in combination with nicotine replacement therapies. It's a great way to keep your mind and body healthy.

Walk this Way . . .

If you think you can't get a great workout from walking, think again! Recent research on walking programs shows that moving at a moderately brisk pace for 45 minutes three times per week at about 60% of your maximum heart rate significantly increased cardiorespiratory fitness and can decrease blood pressure, plasma triglyceride, cholesterol, and low-density lipoprotein (LDL) cholesterol levels, while increasing good high-density lipoprotein (HDL) cholesterol concentrations. Participants also lost body weight, fat stores, and decreased their waist size!

And researchers from Harvard Medical School looking at stroke risk studied almost 40,000 female health professionals. The findings, which were published in 2010 in *Stroke: Journal of the American Heart Association,* showed that women who walked two or more hours a week at about three miles per hour or faster were significantly less likely to suffer a stroke than less active women.

Beyond heart health . . . additional benefits of exercise:

- Decreased anxiety and depression
- Reduced cravings to smoke

- Improved lung function
- Improvements in arthritis
- Improved sleep quality
- Better memory
- Reduced signs of aging
- Improved bone health
- Lower risk of cancer

10,000 Steps a Day–The Key to a Healthy Heart

Pedometers count the number of steps per day and are an inexpensive and effective motivator. Strive to achieve at least 10,000 steps per day.

Purchasing a pedometer (most cost less than $20) that measures the number of steps you take is one of the best investments you can make. Walking 10,000 steps each day is considered to be a goal for daily exercise. Unfortunately, most of us walk less than 3,000 steps per day.

A study published in the *American Journal of Preventive Medicine* found that those who walk 10,000 steps each day reduce their odds of developing metabolic syndrome by 72%. More than one out of three Americans have metabolic syndrome, which increases their risk of heart disease and diabetes and is characterized by having at least three of the following:

- Abdominal obesity

- Elevated level of triglycerides
- Low level of HDL cholesterol
- Elevated blood pressure
- Elevated fasting glucose levels.

Building up to 10,000 steps a day can help control weight and may reduce diabetes risk, suggests research in the *British Medical Journal*.

Of 592 middle-aged Australian adults, those who increased the number of steps they took during a five-year period and built up to 10,000 steps per day had a lower body mass index, less belly fat, and better insulin sensitivity than their counterparts, who did not take as many steps daily during the same time period. This helps to reduce the risk of obesity, diabetes, and heart disease.

Increase your steps per day by:

- Scheduling a 30-to-45 minute walk each day
- Walking during your lunch break
- Walking in place while watching TV
- Using stairs rather than elevators

Where to Start?

Beginning your fitness routine is simple. Aside from picking the activities you enjoy the most, there are essentially three concepts to incorporate in your program:

- how often you plan to exercise (frequency)
- how hard you can exercise (intensity)
- how long you should exercise (time or duration)

To help you remember, the American Heart Association (AHA) created the "FIT Formula" of *frequency, intensity, and time.*

When considering the exercise *frequency* and *time* that will benefit your heart, lungs, and circulation, organizations like the AHA and the American College of Sports Medicine (ACSM) jointly recommend doing moderately intense cardio activities 30 minutes a day, five days a week. Of course, you may need to start slowly if you are more sedentary. Aiming for 20 minutes of exercise three to five times a week is a great goal for the first few weeks. Eventually, you should strive to achieve at least 30 minutes of aerobic activity, like walking, every day.

Intensity refers to how hard you want to work during your exercise. A simple rule of thumb is that you should break a sweat but still be able to carry on a conversation.

Get *FIT (Frequence, Intensity, Time)*
Frequency: 3–5 times per week
Intensity: Break a sweat but able to carry on a conversation
Time: 20–30 minutes

Resistance Training

Resistance training and muscle-strengthening exercises, also called isometric exercise, involve using the muscles to pull or push a weight, even our own bodyweight.

Resistance training promotes lean muscle mass and maintains muscle tone, which may help to efficiently metabolize glucose. In women, research shows that resistance training maintains bone mineral density, helping to ward off osteoporosis. Finally, keeping good muscle tone helps to maintain a healthy weight—lean muscle burns more calories, thereby increasing your resting metabolism.

A study in the March 2019 *Medicine & Science in Sports & Exercise* examined the exercise habits of almost 13,000 adults (average age 47) who did not have cardiovascular disease. This study found that those who did at least an hour per week of weight training (using free weights or weight machines) had a 40% to 70% lower risk of heart attack or stroke compared with those who did not exercise.

What are some good ways to begin resistance training? Your own body weight, resistance bands or pulleys, free weights, medicine balls, or weight machines are all good options. And there is no need to overdo it. Eight resistance exercises at 10 repetitions each is sufficient.

Sample Fitness Plan–Strength/Resistance Training

Exercise	Reps	Muscle Group
Push-ups	10	Chest
Biceps Curls	10	Biceps
Triceps Curls	10	Triceps
Lunges	8–10 each leg	Quadriceps, hamstrings
Overhead Press	10	Shoulders
Sit-ups	12	Abdominals
Rowing	10	Back
Calf raises	12 each side	Gastrocnemius

Caution:

Always check with your personal treating physician prior to starting an exercise program. If you have a history of cardiovascular disease or cardiac risk factors, then your doctor may want you to have a stress test prior to clearing you for an exercise program. In addition, if you are starting a resistance or weight-training program, consider working with a certified personal trainer to get you started.

Are You Ready?

Research shows that we are more likely to create fitness habits when we participate in activities we enjoy, and it makes sense.

A great way to start is by walking (30 to 45 minutes or 10,000 steps per day). If you have the time to enjoy other activities such as tennis, golf (walking), swimming, or biking, then do it! Otherwise, walk, walk, walk—your heart will thank you!

Sample Fitness Plan–Beginner

Mon.	Tues.	Wed.	Thurs.	Friday	Sat.	Sun.
Rest	Walk 30 min	Bike 30 min	Walk 30 min	Rest	Walk 30 min	Walk 30 min

Sample Fitness Plan–Intermediate

Mon.	Tues.	Wed.	Thurs.	Friday	Sat.	Sun.
Walk 30 min	Walk 30 min	Strength train 8–10 exercises, 10 reps	Bike 30 min	Walk 30 min	Walk 30 min	Strength train 8–10 exercises, 8–12 reps

Tip! If you can't squeeze in a continuous 30 minutes of exercise into your day, try breaking up the 30 minutes into three 10-minute intervals. Studies have shown that this will also improve your cardiovascular fitness.

Did You know? A Note on Active Living

In 1997 the CDC (Centers for Disease Control) began the Active Living Initiative, which aims to better understand how our environment can be improved to support more active lifestyles. The initiative is tapping into the expertise of urban planners, architects, engineers, public health experts, and physicians. Active Living as a way of life incorporates physical activity into daily routines, such as walking to the store or biking to work. How active is your living?

Want more information or want to get involved? Visit www.activelivingbydesign.org

Sitting Time and Heart Attack Risk

Reduction of sitting time is an important strategy for preventing heart attacks and premature mortality in physically inactive individuals.

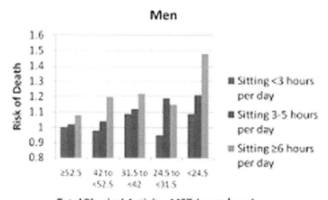

Low risk indicates sitting less than four hours per day. Medium risk indicates sitting four to eight hours per day. High risk indicates sitting eight to eleven hours per day. Very high risk indicates sitting more than 11 hours per day.

People who sit for a large proportion of their working day also report sitting for longer outside work and do not compensate for their sedentary behavior at work by being more active outside work.

Sitting is therefore associated with increased heart attack risk, even in those who exercise outside of work.

Many have suggested that setting an alert on your phone every 50 minutes on the hour to get up and exercise in place for 10 minutes will help to reduce the risk of prolonged sitting.

Key Points

> Get clearance to start an exercise program from your personal treating physician.

> Get a pedometer and strive for 10,000 steps per day.

> Start some form of exercise regularly, whether it's walking, biking, tennis, or swimming.

> Avoid prolonged sitting.

> Regular aerobic exercise improves cardiorespiratory fitness, decreases blood pressure, lowers triglyceride and LDL cholesterol, and increases HDL cholesterol. It also lowers the risk of cardiovascular disease.

➤ Resistance exercise (one hour per week) lowers the risk of heart attack and stroke.

➤ Exercise helps to achieve weight loss and maintain normal body weight. It also helps to reduce harmful visceral or belly fat.

CHAPTER 8

Stress–The Forgotten Risk Factor

Creating a Stress-free Life

Are you a worrier? Or do you have anxiety and toss and turn at night? Do you have a "short fuse?" Are you a "hot reactor?" Or do you hold everything in as long as you can and then explode when others least expect it?

It is important that you understand your stress type, identify your triggers, and learn new ways to manage your stress. By doing so, you can lessen the negative affects stress has on your life and your health.

I have found that many people overlook stress as a risk factor for heart disease, even in the medical community. Each of us perceives stress and stressors differently and thus has a different response. The fact remains that we all experience stress, from the small stuff we're not supposed to sweat— like traffic jams and getting the kids to practice on time—to the big stuff, like being laid off from your job or dealing with a divorce or the passing of a loved one. They're all part of the stress stew.

It's important to know that you are not alone in feeling stress. We all feel it. But some of us have learned skills along the way that make handling it easier. So let's learn how to take the lemons life gives us and make lemonade.

The Stress Response

Our body's ability to perceive and react to stress is actually a good thing—it's an ancient, innate defense mechanism to keep us alive. Remember the fight-or-flight response to stress? It hasn't changed. Early man relied on a sudden surge of hormones to fight off or flee an imminent threat, like a saber-toothed tiger. The problem for modern man is that, while we thankfully don't face off with wild animals anymore, our hormonal responses don't see it that way.

That car that just cut you off, the looming deadline to get the reports in by the end of the day, and the washer breaking down (and how to pay for it) all evoke a stress response. And to our bodies, this may as well have been a lion, tiger, and bear attacking us all in one day.

While ancient man may have confronted 1 or 2 stressful events in a week, today we have 20 to 30 stressful stimuli per day that our brains perceive to be direct threats. Pink slips, financial stressors, and marital strain are just as threatening as the ferocious tiger, and when they occur on a regular basis, they can have an even more deleterious effect. The result is we are living in a constant state of physiological stress.

So what is the stress response, and how does it affect our heart? Stress and anger increase the release of stress hormones, such as adrenaline and cortisol. These have a natural effect of increasing blood pressure, cholesterol, and blood sugar, causing the heartbeat to become rapid and increasing the "stickiness" of our platelets, which increases the likelihood of a blood clot. All of this together is one big red flag for a heart attack or stroke. How you handle daily stress is key to keeping stress hormones, and the stress response, under control.

Heading for a Heartbreak?

The heat wave won't let up, you're late, and there is a massive traffic jam. Sound familiar? Just as soon as you see the open lane to move ahead, a car whips in front of you. You slam on the brakes, lay on the horn, and spout off a wave of expletives. You're going nowhere, but your heart is in overdrive! It is like driving your car at 80 miles per hour with your brakes on—how much stress can your heart take before it says enough?

Decades ago, important research was conducted by the late cardiologist Dr. Robert Elliot. Dr. Elliot determined that people who become angered easily to stressful situations also had extreme cardiovascular responses—their bodies produced large amounts of stress hormones with rapid elevation in blood pressure and heart rate. These so-called hot reactors are quick to react to everyday stimuli, causing the stress response to happen multiple times a day. Hot reactors are at greater risk for developing stress-related cardiovascular conditions such as heart attack and sudden cardiac death.

Hot reactors are different from "Type A" personalities, or the workaholic types who are driven, competitive, and highly demanding of themselves and others. What we've learned is that there is nothing wrong with being driven and ambitious. What really affects us is if we are habitually impatient, hostile, and angry. These are the traits that put us at risk because they activate the stress response through the sympathetic nervous system.

While we may not feel it, our arteries constrict, our platelets get sticky, heart rate and blood pressure skyrockets, and the body shunts blood to the muscles. Quite a physiological reaction!

Hot Reactor Quiz:

- Are you always angry?
- Do you have chronic hostility?
- Do you explode when confronted with stress?
- Do you get red in the face and feel your heart pounding with even the slightest provocation?

If you answered yes to any of the above, you may be a hot reactor.

Keep in mind that you may have none of the classic signs or symptoms of a hot reactor but still have an exaggerated physiologic response to mental stress. Discuss this with your health care provider, as there are ways to diagnose and treat this condition.

Anxiety

While anxiety hasn't traditionally been thought to provoke the same immense stress response as in a hot reactor, new research is showing that anxiety is indeed associated with negative cardiovascular outcomes. In a study published in the *Archives of General Psychiatry*, generalized anxiety disorder was associated with 74% increased risk of a cardiovascular event, including death, in patients with coronary artery disease.

So anxiety is not so great either. What does all of this mean for you? We all have a little hot reactor in us, and we all understand the feeling of anxiety. Minimizing both will boost our happiness quotient and benefit us mentally and physically. No matter who we are, we all can benefit from techniques and methods—from meditation and yoga to simply laughing more—to manage our stress, lighten our load, and overall live happier and healthier lives.

Distressed and Depressed

Fred was a recently divorced father of two teenage boys. In his early 50s, he had led a relatively healthy life. He was active, volunteered in his community, believed in a low-stress life, and had a long, successful career in advertising. Then the economy took a downturn, and magazines, newspapers and periodicals started closing left and right. Fred lost his job. Naturally, he began worrying about how he would take care of his boys; where would he find the money to pay for them to go to college? And then Fred started to become depressed.

I know this because the first time I met Fred was in the hospital. He had suffered a heart attack. He told me how, after he lost his job, he slowly stopped communicating with friends. He lost touch with his former colleagues, many of whom had tried to reach out to him numerous times. He was tired and didn't have the energy to volunteer. And after unsuccessfully vying for several new positions, he felt defeated.

Although different than the hot reactor, isolated, distressed, and depressed individuals are finding themselves at a greater risk for heart disease and sudden cardiac arrest than those who maintain strong support networks and social circles.

This personality type has recently been identified as a Type D—Distressed and Depressed. Type Ds are characterized as identifying with chronic negative emotions, pessimism, and social inhibition.

Researchers at the University of Tilburg in the Netherlands looked at 49 studies of more than 6,000 Type D patients with heart conditions to assess their future heart health and psychological health. What they found was that the chronically down and isolated person was three times more likely to suffer a future cardiovascular event, including heart attack or sudden cardiac death, than a non-Type D person.

A Type D profile was also linked to a three-fold increase in long-term risk of psychological conditions, including clinical depression, anxiety, or poor mental health.

"Type D patients tend to experience increased levels of anxiety, irritation, and depressed mood across situations and time, while not sharing these emotions with others because of fear of disapproval," noted Viola Spek, PhD, a researcher and author of the study, which was published in the American Heart Association journal *Circulation*. "We found that a Type D personality predicts mortality and morbidity in these patients, independent of traditional medical risk factors."

The National Heart, Lung, and Blood Institute and researchers at Indiana University-Purdue University Indianapolis examined the relationship between depression and inflammation in the body. They found that, over time, depressive symptoms are associated with increases in interleukin-6 (IL-6), an inflammatory protein that can predict cardiovascular events.

According to the study, which was published in the journal *Brain, Behavior, and Immunity,* the relationship between depression and future heart disease is similar in strength to well-known risk factors like smoking, high blood pressure, and elevated cholesterol.

If you find you are more of a Type D personality than a Type A, managing stress for you will mean learning to reach out to friends and family more, trying to venture out to meet new people and try new things, and generally stay upbeat and active. Exercise, even moderate walking, is proven to alleviate depression and increase the release of endorphins, or the "feel good" hormones, in the body.

Managing your stress and depression is vital to your survival, especially if you already have underlying heart disease, according to a recent study of approximately 6,000 British citizens who were followed for more than five years. Researchers from Europe and the United States determined that patients with heart disease and depression were five times more likely to die of any cause than those patients with only depression or only heart disease. Therefore, if you suffer from depression, discuss this with your physician and get evaluated and treated by a qualified mental health professional.

Panic Attacks

Anxiety and depression can affect all of us at different times in our lives and for different reasons. Job loss, fear of financial instability in a poor economic climate, life changes, and even small, daily events of life can trigger feelings of helplessness or angst. For some of us, this may take the shape of a panic attack. Sufferers of a panic attack often described them as having an intense feeling of an emergency but without any ability to know what it is or how to respond.

Physical symptoms can follow, including extreme shortness of breath, rapid heartbeat, chest pain, and heightened perception of fear.

Some panic attacks prevent people from going out, being social, or participating in an activity that could be a trigger to anxiety.

If you are prone to panic attacks, have had them in the past, or know someone who has them, there are two points I want to stress.

First, it is important that your physician is aware of your condition since it can be managed with behavioral therapy and medications.

Second, panic attacks may be linked to a higher risk of heart attacks and heart disease, particularly in those 50 or younger, according to new research out of London. Researchers at the University College London looked at data from more than 300,000 individuals and found that people first diagnosed with panic attacks are 33% more likely to have a heart attack compared to those without the condition. In addition, heart disease among study participants with panic symptoms was especially high among women under age 50. The study, published in the *European Heart Journal,* stressed the need to discuss any panic attack symptoms, which can often mimic a heart attack, with your doctor.

Be Social, Stay Connected!

Social isolation can also wreak havoc on your heart. A study from the National Heart, Lung, and Blood Institute suggested that social isolation adversely affected the cardiovascular system by activating the sympathetic nervous system and the hypothalamic-pituitary-adrenal pathways.

Another study analyzed an elderly population. Older men who have few personal relationships have increased risk of heart disease, according to a report presented at the American Heart Association's Scientific Sessions in 2003. In a study examining factors that influence successful aging, researchers found that among a group of men in their 70s, social isolation was linked to increased levels of C-reactive protein (CRP), interleukin-6 (IL-6) and fibrinogen in the blood. These blood components are elevated during inflammation.

Recent research has suggested that inflammation in the body is a risk marker for cardiovascular disease. People with elevated CRP and fibrinogen have higher risks for heart attack and stroke

Therefore, maintaining balance, reducing stress, and having a reliable support network is essential to your health and your survival.

Inhale and Exhale!

An interesting fact about the body is that your mental state is different than your physical state. We can retrain our mind to see that traffic jam, fender bender, or demanding boss as what they are and not a ferocious beast. One of the easiest and simplest things you can do the very first moment you feel stress is to breathe deeply and slowly. In that moment of panic or anxiety, take a deep breath and try to relax.

In contrast to the stress response, breathing calms the body and lowers heart rate and blood pressure. It is also one of the important processes in your body's relaxation response.

Practice the Relaxation Response

Many years ago, Dr. Herbert Benson of Harvard Medical School, and founder of the Mind-Body Institute in Boston, shared with me at my annual heart disease prevention symposium a revolutionary way to manage stress. He identified the steps in the relaxation response and put them into deliberate practice. Today, I recommend this easy, step-by-step process to all of my patients. It only takes 10–15 minutes and does wonders for minimizing stress and your body's response to it.

The Relaxation Response:

1. Sit quietly in a comfortable position.
2. Close your eyes and visualize each muscle relaxing, beginning with your feet, moving up through your thighs, all the way up to your back, neck, arms, and hands, and up to your face. **Let go of any tension, and** let your muscles remain relaxed.
3. Breathe deeply and slowly, bringing your attention to your breath and how your chest rises and falls with each inhale and exhale.
4. When you are comfortable, choose a word that represents relaxation to you. Perhaps it is "peace" or "calm," and say it to yourself with each inhalation.
5. Continue for about 10 minutes or as long as you feel comfortable. Allow yourself to sit quietly for several minutes, **reawakening your senses a bit,** and don't feel pressure to stand until you are alert.

Congratulations! You've just learned a wonderful skill you can use to manage your stress, anytime and almost anywhere. You can turn to breathing whenever you need it.

You will rely on focused breathing as the anchor to any other relaxation technique you choose, whether it's meditation, yoga, or exercise.

Meditation

Meditation builds on the process of the relaxation response by adding imagery, additional words or sayings, sounds, or symbols. Some may think meditation is too alternative or existential. But really it can be whatever you want it to be. These are ancient techniques, traced back some five thousand years and possibly earlier, but the purpose of meditation is to allow the body to relax and the mind to focus on something positive in the here and now.

Meditation also has a positive effect on the cardiovascular system! One meditative practice you may have heard of is transcendental meditation. This technique is similar to the relaxation response. It can be practiced twice per day for 20 minutes with eyes closed and involves the use of a mantra or specific saying. In a study of two hundred African American patients with coronary heart disease, those who practiced the meditation technique had almost 50% lower rates of heart attack, stroke, and death compared to non-meditating patients who were simply given educational information about their condition.

In addition, patients who meditated saw their blood pressure drop. Researchers at The Medical

College of Wisconsin also found that participants perceived their stress levels to be significantly less than prior to the study.

You don't have to practice transcendental meditation to achieve these same results. The message is just to incorporate relaxation time in your day with the technique you like most.

Meditation also provides many other benefits, as now proven in many research studies. For example, meditation has been shown to:

- improve one's ability to manage pain
- improve one's ability to manage anger
- improve one's cognitive abilities
- increase attention span

Yoga

The benefits of yoga for the mind and the body can also be traced back some five thousand years to India and other Eastern civilizations. In the last few years, yoga has become increasingly popular, moving from an alternative type of exercise to one that is offered at almost every gym in the country and practiced by athletes and those seeking a stress-free life alike. Several studies have shown that yoga can lower cholesterol and triglycerides, lower blood pressure, and reduce cardiometabolic risk factors.

Simply translated as "union," yoga in the traditional sense connects the body with the spirit for the goal of achieving peace, physical and mental balance, and well-being.

Relying on deep breathing as the foundation of its practice, yoga is based on hundreds of specific poses, or asanas, each designed to promote relaxation, balance, flexibility, and strength. Because yoga is noncompetitive, it promotes self-acceptance, listening to your body and mind, concentration, and is suitable for all ages.

Because yoga has become more popular, it has also become the subject of research studies. If you have ever practiced yoga, you probably won't be surprised to learn that the research is positive. Yoga can improve many conditions, from depression and anxiety to pain and asthma, and yes, cardiovascular conditions.

Ohio State University researchers just reported in the journal *Psychosomatic Medicine* results from a study showing that women who routinely practiced yoga had lower amounts of the inflammatory marker, interleukin-6 (IL-6) in their blood than non-practicing women. The practicing women also showed smaller increases of IL-6 after undergoing stressful experiences than women who were the same age and weight but who were not yoga practitioners. IL-6 is an important part of the body's inflammatory response and has been shown to be a biomarker in heart disease, stroke, type-2 diabetes, arthritis, and other inflammatory and age-related diseases.

The study also measured C-reactive protein (CRP), another key inflammatory marker discussed earlier, as part of your comprehensive blood test. What the researchers found was that women who did not practice yoga regularly had CRP levels 4.75 times higher than the women who regularly engaged in the mind-body exercise.

Another study out of Boston University's School of Medicine identified that a yoga session increased the level of gamma-aminobutyric acid (GABA), a chemical that is reduced in people with mood and anxiety disorders. Increased GABA levels after a yoga session are associated with improved mood and decreased anxiety, more so than the increases seen after moderate exercise, the scientists said.

Asanas for Stress

One of the easiest ways to experience yoga and begin to incorporate it into your life is to take a class. If you belong to a gym, check to see if they have yoga offerings. Typical class names include Yoga Flow, Vinyasa Yoga, Hatha Yoga, etc. As mentioned, because yoga is noncompetitive, almost all classes will welcome beginners, except perhaps a Power Yoga class, which is designed for those with considerable strength and cardiovascular fitness.

In yoga, there are various poses or asanas that are specifically designed to calm the mind and nervous system. Practicing these poses regularly or when you feel stressed can greatly relieve tension and anxiety.

As with any new physical activity, be sure to check with your doctor before starting.

Laughter and Living Well

There's a final note I'd like to make about managing your stress. There is simply nothing better for mood, stress release, and overall well-being than a good, deep laugh. Children laugh on average about three hundred times per day. Adults? About 15 times—if we're lucky. We need to remember how good it feels to laugh and how beneficial it can be to our health. Laughter may very well be the best medicine.

I have noticed that over the years that my patients who seemed to laugh more, took things in stride, and found a piece of humor in even the most stressful news had fewer heart attacks and lived longer.

And I've come across study after study that identifies ways laughter promotes a beneficial and "feel-good" response in the body, and specifically improves cardiovascular health. Research has found that laughter decreases the hormone cortisol, thereby lowering heart attack risk.

Laughter even seems to affect the blood vessels themselves. Research done at the cardiology department of Athens Medical School found that laughter improved arterial stiffness in healthy individuals. Similarly, studies at the University of Maryland

Medical Center in Baltimore suggest that laughing may be as beneficial as exercise in relaxing arteries and increasing blood flow.

And some scientists have hypothesized that laughter releases chemicals that are protective to the artery lining, preventing cholesterol from entering the wall to form the plaques that cause heart attack. Michael Miller, MD, director of the University of Maryland's center for preventative cardiology, has said, "Because we know many more factors that contribute to heart disease than factors that protect against it, the ability to laugh—either naturally or as a learned behavior—may have important implications in certain societies such as the United States, where heart disease remains the number one killer. Thirty minutes of exercise three times a week and fifteen minutes of hearty laughter each day should be part of a healthy lifestyle."

When you think about it, laughter is wonderful! The mere expectation of laughing, or seeing a comedic movie, or telling a funny joke, makes us feel good. An interesting study split a group of sixteen people into two groups. One group was told they would be watching a funny movie and the other group (the control group) would not. Blood was drawn from all subjects just before the video was started. The subjects who were told they were going to see a funny movie had 27% more beta-endorphins (the feel-good hormone) in their blood sample than those subjects in the control group.

The elevated levels of beta-endorphins remained elevated in the group during the video and continued to be elevated for 12–24 hours afterward. It was concluded that these results, combined with other research on how laughter improves mood, are proof positive of just how good a hearty chuckle is for your wellness, disease prevention, and stress reduction.

In Austria, "laughter yoga," a mix of breathing, laughing, and stretching, has improved the recovery and well-being of stroke victims at Graz University, and may significantly lower blood pressure.

Who doesn't feel relaxed, calm, and happy after a good bought of laughter? Often in our stressful lives, we forget to embrace the things we can do naturally to bring joy into our world. Laughing is a physiologic response, just like coughing or crying. But we must remember to use it.

FACT! There are more than 6,000 laughter clubs in 60 countries.

Key Points

> Chronic stress leads to elevated blood pressure, increased heart rate, inflammation, oxidative stress, poor sleep quality, insulin resistance and diabetes.

> Chronic stress significantly increases the risk of cardiovascular disease, including heart attack and stroke.

➢ Reducing stress lowers cardiovascular risk.

➢ For those who have stress despite healthy lifestyle choices, medical and behavioral therapy has been shown to be beneficial.

➢ Holistic approach for stress control:

  ➢ Regular exercise

  ➢ Relax after meals

  ➢ Meditation

  ➢ Prayer

  ➢ Yoga

  ➢ Relaxation response

  ➢ Mindfulness

  ➢ Close relationship with family and friends

  ➢ Set realistic goals in life

  ➢ Live within your means

  ➢ Have a positive outlook in life

  ➢ Never lose your sense of humor

  ➢ Laugh, smile, and enjoy life

CHAPTER 9

Smoking and Air Pollution–Risk Factors to be Eliminated

Smoking: Kick the habit.

If you smoke—commit to quit! Make that commitment to yourself and your loved ones. Quitting is critical to making yourself heart healthy. In addition, cigarette smoking can cause cancer almost anywhere in the body. Smoking has been known to cause cancer of the mouth, throat, esophagus, lung, stomach, colon, rectum, liver, pancreas, larynx, trachea, bronchus, kidney, bladder, and cervix. Cigarette smoking is also the leading cause of chronic obstructive pulmonary disease, including emphysema and chronic bronchitis.

If you don't smoke or have already quit, congratulations! You are making one of the best decisions of your life.

Those who smoke are two-to-three times more likely to die from coronary heart disease than non-smokers. And each additional cigarette you smoke per day increases your risk. Smoking just one to four cigarettes per day equates to almost a three-fold higher risk of dying from coronary heart disease compared with not smoking.

And once you quit, your risk of heart disease and stroke will decrease, no matter how long you have smoked or how much you have smoked over your lifetime—even if you've been a heavy smoker! Studies show that your cardiovascular risk will significantly decrease within the first two years of smoking cessation.

Data showing just how much you can protect yourself from dying from a heart attack if you stop smoking are overwhelming, even if you have already suffered one. Israeli Professor Yaacov Drory recently examined this in research published in the *The Journal of the American College of Cardiology*. What Professor Drory found was that quitting smoking after a heart attack was almost as effective as other approaches, including invasive procedures and statins or lipid-lowering drugs. Professor Drory's data spanned more than 13 years, and even after accounting for lifestyle, socioeconomic, and other cardiovascular factors (like exercise and obesity), still found that quitting smoking was the most important risk-factor modification linked to long-term survival. Specifically, compared to patients who continued to smoke, those who quit smoking before their first heart attack had a 50% lower mortality rate, while those who quit after their first heart attack still benefited by lowering their risk by 37%.

Begin a smoke-free life. No, it is not always easy. But the good news is that there are new and better ways to help you quit, such as behavioral therapy and medications. Discuss your optimal smoking cessation approach with your health care provider.

Smokeless Tobacco-Users Beware

So you don't smoke cigarettes. Good. But do you use smokeless tobacco products like snuff and chewing tobacco, thinking they are healthier than lighting up? Think again. Multiple research studies conducted over the last 30 years have shown the opposite. Professors at the International Agency for Cancer Research in France analyzed data from over 11 studies conducted in Europe and North America and found that, in fact, smokeless tobacco does increase your risk of dying from a heart attack or stroke.

For those who are unable to quit smoking on their own, a combination of medications and socially supportive counseling has always seemed to work best. One great place to start is the internet. There are many web-based support groups, including smoke-free.gov, that can help you on your path to a smoke-free life.

Smoking Cessation Tips

- If you can quit "cold turkey," then do so. If not, then each day, smoke fewer and fewer cigarettes until you wean yourself off completely.

- Carry sugarless gum with you, and munch on finger-food snacks, like carrots, celery, and apple sticks.
- Stay busy, manage your stress, and drink lots of water.
- Begin a regular walking program.
- Know your triggers! They are often why earnest attempts to quit fail.
- Don't beat yourself up! Stay positive. You will succeed.

How about vaping or e-cigarettes? They are also unhealthy and significantly increase the risk of heart attack and stroke. It was reported in 2019 that compared with nonusers, people who use e-cigarettes have a 71% higher risk of stroke and a 59% higher risk of heart attack or angina. In addition, those who smoke e-cigarettes are more likely to switch to regular cigarettes.

Don't forget to also avoid "secondhand" or passive smoking by being near those who smoke. Nonsmokers who are exposed to secondhand smoke at home or at work increase their risk of developing heart disease by 25%–30%. Secondhand smoke increases the risk for stroke by 20%–30%.

Finally, avoid exposure to air pollution. Chronic air pollution leads to more than three million deaths worldwide each year. It increases the risk of heart attack, stroke, high blood pressure, irregular heart rhythm, chronic obstructive lung disease, and cancer.

Key Points

> Cigarette smoking significantly increases the risk of heart attack and stroke.

> Vaping and e-cigarette smoking also increases the risk of heart attack and stroke.

> Cigarette smoking increases the risk of cancer and chronic obstructive pulmonary disease, including emphysema and chronic bronchitis.

> Behavioral therapy and medications can help you quit smoking if you are unable to quit on your own.

> Avoid chronic exposure to secondhand or passive smoking since it can significantly increase the risk of heart attack and stroke.

> Avoid chronic exposure to air pollution—it increases the risk of heart attack, stroke, high blood pressure, irregular heart rhythm, lung disease and cancer.

CHAPTER 10

Sleep Quality and Heart Health

Napping and Sleep Quality

Clinical studies have supported the benefits of a midday nap. A large study found that people who regularly took a siesta were significantly less likely to die of heart disease.

"Taking a nap could turn out to be an important weapon in the fight against coronary mortality," said Dimitrios Trichopoulos of the Harvard School of Public Health in Boston, who led the study published in the Archives of Internal Medicine.

The study of more than 23,000 Greek adults found that those who regularly took a midday nap were more than 30% less likely to die of heart disease.

The truth is, napping reduces stress. It is natural to feel drowsy in the afternoon, and research has shown that a brief nap can result in greater alertness, reduced levels of stress, and improved cognitive function. And many adults understandably experience a natural decrease in alertness after six to eight hours of working, especially if they don't get enough nighttime sleep. But for some reason, our culture frowns on the idea that midday naps are beneficial for anyone other than small children or the elderly. Research tells us otherwise.

Midday napping, or a short siesta, is common in populations with low rates of death from coronary heart disease.

Napping also improves your mental and cognitive abilities. A NASA study showed that a short nap boosted airline pilots' performance by 33%. In fact, a midday catnap can recharge your batteries better than drinking a cup of coffee, and studies show that people who power nap get better results on memory tests than those who drink caffeine.

So what's considered a power nap? A 15–30-minute nap in the afternoon seems to provide significant health benefits—though most experts feel that napping more than 30 minutes puts you into a deeper stage of sleep and makes it more difficult for you to fall asleep at night.

Nightime Sleep

Most of us need about seven hours of sleep a night. Sleep quality and quantity affects your risk of diseases, including diabetes and heart disease. Data coming out of the West Virginia University School of Medicine are pointing to a direct relationship between sleep time—both too short and too long—and cardiovascular disease.

When researchers looked at the sleep patterns and other demographic and lifestyle characteristics of 30,397 adults who participated in the 2005 National Health Interview Survey, they found that people who reported sleeping less than five hours per night were twice as likely to develop any cardiovascular disease compared to those who slept seven hours. Interestingly, those who slept nine hours or more also had an increased risk of developing cardiovascular disease, even after accounting for factors that might otherwise influence the results, such as age, sex, race, smoking, alcohol consumption, body mass index, physical activity, diabetes, hypertension, and depression.

According to the authors of the study, which was published in the journal *SLEEP*, the mechanisms underlying the association between short sleep and cardiovascular disease may include sleep-related disturbances in endocrine and metabolic functions, including impaired glucose tolerance, reduced insulin sensitivity, increased sympathetic activity, and elevated blood pressure, all of which increase the risk of heart attack and stroke.

Similarly, researchers from the University of Warwick and the State University of New York at Buffalo discovered that people who sleep less than six hours per night may be three times more likely to find themselves in a pre-diabetic state called impaired fasting glucose (IFG). People with IFG are typically at a greater risk for developing type 2 diabetes because they cannot regulate their glucose levels as well as a healthy person can, which can also lead to an increased risk of heart disease and stroke.

A similar study looked at sleep loss and insulin resistance in healthy people. What the researchers found was alarming. Just one night of sleeping about four hours induced insulin resistance in healthy adults, according to researchers at the Leiden University Medical Center in The Netherlands and results published in the *Journal of Clinical Endocrinology & Metabolism.*

Inadequate sleep has also been associated with increased consumption of sweet and fatty foods due to an increase in the body of the hunger hormone ghrelin. As a result, sleep deprivation is associated with an increased risk of obesity.

Sleep Apnea–The Often-Unrecognized Risk Factor for Heart Attack and Stroke

The nighttime breathing disorder known as obstructive sleep apnea increases a person's risk of having a heart attack or dying by 30% over a period of four to five years, according to a recent study.

The study found that the more severe the sleep apnea, the greater the risk of developing heart disease or dying.

"While previous studies have shown an association between sleep apnea and heart disease, ours is a large study that allowed us to not only follow patients for five years and look at the association between sleep apnea and the combined outcome of heart attack and death, but also adjust for other traditional risk factors for heart disease," says researcher Neomi Shah, MD, of Yale University. Shah went on to say, "there is some evidence to make us believe that when sleep apnea is appropriately treated, the risk of heart disease can be lowered."

In obstructive sleep apnea, the upper airway narrows, or collapses, during sleep. Periods of apnea end with a brief partial arousal that may disrupt sleep hundreds of times a night. Obesity is a major risk factor for sleep apnea.

If left untreated, sleep apnea can lead to hypertension, atrial fibrillation (a heart rhythm disorder), heart attack, and stroke.

The most effective treatment for sleep apnea is a technique called CPAP, for continuous positive airway pressure, which delivers air through a mask while the patient sleeps, keeping the airway open. It has proved successful in many cases in providing a good night's sleep, preventing daytime accidents due to sleepiness, and improving quality of life.

Sleep apnea triggers the body's fight-or-flight mechanism, discussed earlier, which increases the risk of heart attack. In addition, episodes of apnea or breathing cessation results in oxygen desaturation in the bloodstream.

The signs and symptoms of obstructive sleep apnea include snoring, periods of apnea (breathing cessation) during the night, daytime fatigue or drowsiness, irritability, morning headaches, and memory loss. The diagnosis of sleep apnea is made by conducting a formal sleep study. Treatment includes lifestyle changes, surgery, or CPAP (continuous positive airway pressure) via a mask worn at night.

The message is clear: if you have signs or symptoms of sleep apnea, notify your physician, as effective treatment is available. Early recognition and management may lower your risk of a heart attack or stroke.

Key Points

> Strive to maintain six to eight hours of quality sleep every twenty-four hours.

> Less than six hours of sleep per night increases risk of insulin resistance, diabetes, heart attack, and stroke.

> A regular midday nap lowers the risk of heart disease.

> Obstructive sleep apnea is often associated with snoring during sleep and can lead to daytime fatigue, high blood pressure, headache, atrial fibrillation, heart attack, and stroke.

> Physicians who specialize in sleep disorders can treat poor-quality sleep or sleep apnea and lower the risk of cardiovascular disease.

CHAPTER 11

Diabetes Prevention and Management to Reduce Heart Disease Risk

Blood Sugar and Insulin Resistance

When you went to the doctor, they likely tested your blood sugar to check for diabetes. When we eat, carbohydrates in the food are broken down and enter the bloodstream as glucose to supply our bodies with energy. But glucose levels in the body need to be regulated, which is done by the release of insulin from the pancreas. Normal fasting glucose levels are less than 100 mg/dl, impaired fasting glucose is 100 to 125 mg/dl, and diabetes fasting glucose is greater than 125 mg/dl.

Symptoms from diabetes may include increased thirst, increased hunger, weight loss or gain, frequent urination, fatigue or exhaustion, delayed healing of cuts or sores, and blurred vision.

There are three main types of diabetes:

- Type 1 diabetes, which usually appears in childhood or adolescence, is characterized by a defect in the cells of the pancreas that manufacture insulin. This type of diabetes is generally believed to be related to autoimmune factors or possibly a virus.

- Type 2 diabetes, which usually appears in adults, is caused by insulin resistance (in which cells become resistant or less responsive to insulin). This type of diabetes had been increasing worldwide and is believed to be caused by poor diet and nutrition, lack of exercise, and weight gain.

- Gestational diabetes usually appears during pregnancy and resolves after birth. It does require active monitoring, however, for the safety of the mother and the baby.

Why is insulin so important?

Insulin is a hormone produced by specialized cells in the pancreas and plays a crucial role in allowing our cells to process sugar. In essence, insulin works like a key, "unlocking" cells and allowing glucose to go inside, where it can be used as an energy source or stored as glycogen. Without insulin, glucose remains in the bloodstream, and cells aren't able to receive the energy they need to survive and perform the necessary functions in our body.

In the case of type 2 diabetes, it's as if someone gummed up the locks, so the key no longer fits or works to open up the cells to receive the glucose. In time, the cells that produce the insulin burn out. The result is excessive rises in blood sugar.

When the cells are not able to get the sugar they need to survive, they turn to other sources for energy—such as fatty acids. In addition, elevated blood glucose levels can lead to *advanced glycation end products*, or AGEs, in the blood vessel wall. These AGEs in the walls stimulate the inflammatory cells to release proteinases, which can weaken the fibrous cap of atherosclerotic plaques, leading to rupture and, yes, a heart attack.

The landmark EAST—WEST study showed that diabetic patients without a history of heart attack had the same risk of a future heart attack as those patients without diabetes who had a heart attack. Diabetes is therefore considered a coronary heart disease—risk equivalent. This means that diabetics should be treated as aggressively as non-diabetes with coronary heart disease to prevent future heart attacks.

It is important to maintain a normal blood sugar through good nutrition and regular exercise. The Mediterranean diet was selected as the 2020 best overall diet as well as the best diet to control and prevent diabetes by the US News and World Report. The Mediterranean diet consists of healthy non-processed foods that are rich in fiber and have a low glycemic index—both factors that help to control blood sugar. In addition, this dietary plan does not include refined sugar or starch, which is important for those wishing to prevent diabetes.

Metabolic Syndrome

Metabolic syndrome is increasing in frequency in the United States and around the world due to rising obesity rates and a sedentary lifestyle. Presently, one in four Americans has metabolic syndrome.

When you have three of the following five conditions, you are diagnosed with metabolic syndrome.

1. Abdominal obesity (waist size >40 inches for men and >35 inches for women.
2. High fasting glucose levels (>100 mg/dl)
3. High blood pressure (>130/85 mmHg)
4. Elevated triglycerides (>150 mg/dl)
5. Low HDL (good) cholesterol (<40 for men and <50 for women)

Why should we strive to prevent this? The answer is simple: these conditions can lead to premature heart attacks, strokes, and vascular disease. It has been shown in clinical trials that metabolic syndrome significantly elevates heart attack risk.

New diabetes medications lower heart disease risk

There has been significant progress in the pharmaceutical therapy of diabetes. The most recent medications, SGLT2 inhibitors and the GLP-1 receptor agonists, have been shown to reduce the risk of atherosclerotic coronary heart disease and heart failure, in addition to blood sugar control. These medications represent significant progress in our quest to control blood sugar in diabetes as well as lower the risk of heart attack and heart failure in these patients who are at increased risk of cardiovascular disease. In addition, as compared to prior medications used in the treatment of diabetes, these medications lead to weight loss rather than weight gain.

SGLT2 inhibitors:

- canagliflozin (Invokana)
- dapagliflozin (Farxiga)
- empagliflozin (Jardiance)

GLP-1 receptor agonists:

- Dulaglutide (Trulicity)
- Exenatide (Byetta)
- Liraglutide (Victoza)

Key Points

➢ Diabetes is a coronary heart disease–risk equivalent.

➢ A healthy diet, regular exercise, and maintaining normal body weight is the best way to prevent and treat insulin resistance, pre-diabetes, and diabetes.

> In patients with diabetes, LDL cholesterol should be maintained less than 70 mg/dl with diet, exercise, and cholesterol-lowering medications as needed.

> Triglycerides are often elevated in diabetes, and levels should be maintained less than 150 mg/dl with diet, exercise, and medications as needed.

> Sugar, refined starches, saturated fat, and trans fat should be avoided.

> New medications (SGLT2 inhibitors and GLP agonists) lower blood glucose in diabetics and reduce the risk of cardiovascular disease and heart failure.

CHAPTER 12

Inflammation and Heart Disease

Putting Out the Fires–Lower Inflammation

What many of us don't know is that an unhealthy diet and lifestyle can make inflammation burn like a wildfire in our body. So how does this inflammation affect the heart? Cholesterol trapped in the artery wall will be oxidized by harmful molecules called free radicals. Once that happens, the immune system sends inflammatory cells to attack. This response is what causes a plaque to form, as white blood cells (macrophages) surround and engulf the oxidized cholesterol, which is perceived by the body as a foreign invader.

Major landmark clinical trials have documented that lowering inflammation reduces cardiovascular disease risk. Using high-sensitivity C-reactive protein (hs-CRP) as a marker for vascular inflammation, Dr. Paul Ridker and colleagues showed in the JUPITER TRIAL that healthy men and women without elevated cholesterol but with increased hs-CRP were able to reduce inflammation and major adverse cardiovascular events with a statin (rosuvastatin). In a second trial, CANTOS, Dr. Ridker and colleagues concluded that the addition of anti-inflammatory therapy to cholesterol-lowering therapy in patients with a prior heart attack led to a significantly lower rate of recurrent cardiovascular events. In addition, two recent clinical trials (COLCOT and LODOCO2) showed that low-dose colchicine, an anti-inflammatory medication often used to treat gout, significantly lowered the risk of cardiovascular death, heart attack, and stroke in patients with acute and chronic coronary heart disease.

The more pronounced your body's inflammatory response, the more likely your plaques will rupture and cause dangerous blood clots to form that lead to heart attacks. Why is this? Because inflammatory cells release proteinases that break down the plaque's protective fibrous cap, and they also produce tissue factor that causes blood to clot.

Chronic inflammation may also inhibit the release of nitric oxide, the chemical responsible for the dilation of blood vessels, leading to narrowed arteries, decreased blood flow, and increased blood pressure.

Your heart and cardiovascular system is not the only part of you that is negatively affected by chronic inflammation, however. Swedish scientists have identified that chronic inflammation in the body may contribute to decreased cognitive skills and premature death. Researchers at the Karolinska Institute in Stockholm reported in *Brain, Behavior, and Immunity* that when they studied large population-based registers in more than fifty thousand young men, those with low-grade inflammation performed more poorly on standardized intelligence tests and were more likely to die from a premature death. What is clear is that any inflammatory state that becomes chronic, even on a low-grade level, is hazardous to our health. Indeed, most people don't realize that chronic bronchitis, prostatitis, periodontal disease, obesity, and arthritis all contribute to chronic inflammation. Doing your best to reduce the cause of the inflammation is important to protecting your heart.

It is best to control and manage chronic inflammatory conditions with a healthy diet, regular exercise, and medications when necessary.

What are the causes of chronic inflammation?

Inflammatory Culprit #1–Western Food

The typical American diet—one that is high in red meat, omega-6 fats, trans fat, and refined sugar—actually promotes inflammation. These foods activate chemical pathways that cause a chronic inflammatory state in the body. Unfortunately, the typical American diet is also reliant on packaged and processed foods that are high in fats and sugars, leading us down the road to obesity. This contributes greatly to a state of chronic low-grade inflammation. Fat (adipose) cells release inflammatory proteins into the bloodstream, which increase the risk of cardiovascular disease.

In contrast to a typical American or Western diet, which is pro-inflammatory, a Mediterranean diet is anti-inflammatory. In fact, cold-water omega-3-rich fish, which is commonly consumed in a Mediterranean diet, lowers inflammation, thereby contributing to the health benefits of this dietary eating pattern.

Essentially, what we've learned is that inflammation is involved in all stages of coronary artery disease, from the point at which the plaque forms in the artery wall, to the plaque's progression and rupture, to the clot that blocks blood flow to the heart muscle, resulting in a heart attack.

The best news is that this state of inflammation is reversible with sensible and realistic diet and lifestyle changes. In addition, see your doctor for appropriate medical therapy if you have chronic inflammatory conditions such as arthritis, bronchitis, periodontal disease, prostatitis, inflammatory bowel disease, and autoimmune disease.

Inflammatory Culprit #2–Environmental Toxins

We may not realize it, but our bodies are exposed to numerous microscopic toxins every day. Over time, products like pesticides, chemicals, food additives, and pollution can take their toll, causing our bodies to react in a defensive way by mounting an inflammatory response. Countless epidemiologic studies have found that farmers, migrant workers, and pesticide handlers show increased biomarkers of inflammation, airway inflammation, and asthma. And researchers are finding that environmental concentrations of certain pesticides and insecticides are powerful enough to create conditions like cardiovascular disease.

Indeed, researchers are linking environmental pollution to adverse cardiac outcomes, like heart attacks. A significant study published in the *New England Journal of Medicine* looked at cardiovascular events based on exposure to air pollutants in more than 65,000 postmenopausal women who lived in 36 metropolitan areas in the U.S. The results were conclusive: every incremental rise in particulate matter (10 micrograms per cubic meter) correlated to a 24% increased risk of death from cardiovascular disease.

In Mexico City, where air quality is among the worst of cities in North America, researchers conducted a postmortem study of the hearts of 21 young adults from ages 13–23 from two different areas of the city. What they found was alarming. The young hearts showed signs of chronic inflammation from exposure to particulate matter—pollution found in smoke and haze—as well as endotoxins, or microscopic particles of dead bacteria that attach to particulate matter and gain entry to the body.

A similar study from Long Island Jewish Medical Center compared 24-hour particulate matter counts in New York City to the number of out-of-hospital cardiac arrests. The researchers published in the *American Journal of Epidemiology* that, in fact, on the days when there were rises in small particle air pollution (but still within "safe" levels as determined by the EPA), there was a 4%–10% increase in the number of heart attacks.

And scientists in Germany found that people who live in urban areas where particulate air pollution is high have higher blood pressure than people who live in less polluted areas. In fact, recent studies have linked air pollution to atherosclerosis.

Researchers in Boston conducted a study to assess whether particulates in haze, smog, and smoke affected diabetes. The results, published in *Diabetes Care*, were the first ever to show a correlation between adult diabetes and air pollution, even after accounting for risk factors such as obesity, exercise, and ethnicity. For every incremental rise in pollution, there was a consistent rise in the prevalence of diabetes.

What is interesting about all of these studies is that they have been conducted all over the world and are finding similar results. While it isn't reasonable to expect you or your family members to pack up and move away from your urban condo or your house near the highway, it is useful to realize that these environmental pollutants are affecting our health.

What should you do? Be smart, monitor the air quality in your area, and avoid exercising outdoors when there is an air quality warning. Avoid contact with pesticides and pollutants. Become active in your community to ensure optimal air quality.

Inflammatory Culprit #3–Pro-Inflammatory Disease

There are numerous pro-inflammatory diseases that contribute to chronic inflammation and increase the risk of cardiovascular disease. Examples are arthritis, bronchitis, periodontitis, prostatitis, and inflammatory bowel disease. It is important to seek proper treatment for these conditions.

What About Anti-Inflammatory Medicines?

Certain medications that reduce chronic inflammation have been shown to reduce the risk of heart attack. Aspirin is an excellent example: besides blocking platelets and lowering the risk of blood clots, it also reduces inflammation by targeting and deactivating specific pro-inflammatory enzymes. Statin medications, which are used to lower cholesterol, also reduce inflammation, which further lowers heart attack risk.

A word of caution, however—certain anti-inflammatory medications can also have adverse cardiovascular side effects, such as raising blood pressure and increasing the risk of heart attack. They can also increase the risk of bleeding. This includes many over-the-counter anti-inflammatory medications listed as NSAIDs (nonsteroidal anti-inflammatory

drugs), such as ibuprofen. Although anti-inflammatory medications are sometimes needed, the optimal way to control chronic inflammation is with
a healthy lifestyle. Always discuss the potential
risks of anti-inflammatory medications with your
personal treating physician, and try to avoid the
chronic use of these drugs.

Understanding Free Radicals, Oxidative Stress, and Inflammation

There has been much talk in recent years about the
danger of free radicals. In chemistry, "free radical"
is the term used for any molecule with an uneven
number of electrons. If you remember anything from
chemistry class, it is that molecules with uneven
numbers of electrons don't like to stay that way. And
they'll do whatever they can to beg, borrow, and
steal another electron to have an even number. This
theft by free radicals is referred to as *oxidation.*

Now, it's important to know that oxidation, and
oxidative stress, is essential to living. We need
oxygen to breath to survive, and so do our cells.
Through a process called *cellular respiration,* oxygen turns the food we eat into the energy we need
to live. Cellular respiration is a pretty efficient and
organized process, but it does produce an untow-
ard byproduct in *oxygen free radicals.*

And when oxidation occurs, even though it
is necessary for the survival of our cells, some

damage occurs. A good visual example of this is when you slice an apple. When the apple sits out on the counter, interacting with oxygen in the air, it becomes brown. This is because it is oxidizing and undergoing some damage. The same thing happens inside our bodies, causing tissue damage at the cellular level that can impact our DNA.

In coronary heart disease, cholesterol particles in the bloodstream tend to squeeze through the barrier of endothelial cells and into the artery wall. Once inside the artery wall, cholesterol comes into contact with naturally occurring free radicals. Guess what? They want to steal an electron to feel balanced, and the cholesterol particle has it to give, so the cholesterol becomes oxidized.

Just like with any theft, an alarm is sent out. The body reacts with an immune response, sending inflammatory cells to attack the oxidized cholesterol as if it were a foreign invader. It is this inflammatory immune response that then leads to the development of plaques that progress and rupture, causing clots and eventual heart attacks.

The bad news is that cholesterol isn't the only thing free radicals steal from. Free radicals cause damage on the cellular level in every part of the body. They've been shown to play a part in everything from heart disease to premature aging. And when free radicals steal electrons from DNA, the process leads to abnormal cell behavior and cancer.

What is very important to note is that external toxins and foods can cause free radical production. For example, when toxins enter our bodies, they cause free radical production to go into overdrive. Scientists do not know exactly why this happens, but what we do know is adding noxious and unhealthy items to our body, whether through the environment, smoking, or our food, is like adding lighter fluid to a fire. The result is a free radical explosion.

Free Radical-Producing Toxins

It is impossible to get away from all toxins altogether, but certain offenders are particularly important to be aware of, as they result in extreme free radical production.

Toxins to Avoid

- Air pollutants
- Cigarette smoke
- Excess ultraviolet rays from the sun
- Pesticides
- Radiation (especially CAT scans—unless medically needed)
- Excessive alcohol
- Preservatives in foods and food packaging
- Industrial chemicals
- Household cleaners

- Certain plastics
- Fire retardants

Here's excellent news, however: We know how to fight free radicals. As with many of the risk factors related to heart disease, almost *every single one* can be reversed or reduced through smart and healthy lifestyle choices. We can abstain from smoking (including choosing not to sit close to others who smoke), minimize our exposure to air pollution, and most importantly, avoid the highly processed, calorie-dense, and nutrient-depleted toxic American diet that leads to free radical production.

Do you want to create armies of damaging molecules inside your body simply because you are craving trans fat–rich French fries? Probably not. Would you still want it if you knew that simply changing the food choices could create armies of helpful, beneficial molecules inside your body?

We have a way to make free radicals stable and stop the chain reaction of free radical production. That solution is *antioxidants.*

Antioxidants are the Antidote

We've heard so much in the last few years about antioxidants and their abilities to transform our health for the better. What do they do, and what's their benefit?

How Antioxidants Work

Antioxidants—which include vitamins and nutrients—work by supplying free radicals with the extra electron they would otherwise steal from cholesterol or DNA or other cells. Antioxidants, however, can lose an electron to a free radical without becoming free radicals themselves.

We need thousands of different antioxidants in order for our body to remain healthy. Antioxidants are the body's defense system—they combat and quench the biochemical fires that result from free radical formation. The best way to ensure this happens is to eat a wide range of fruits and vegetables, in a variety of colors, as the different food colors bring a wide variety of free radical–fighting antioxidants to the table.

Some of the various antioxidant-rich fruits and vegetables include:

- Oranges
- Carrots
- Blueberries
- Grapes
- Pomegranates
- Sweet potatoes
- Beets

- Tomatoes
- Garlic
- Broccoli
- Brussels sprouts
- Asparagus
- Spinach

Tap into the Power of these Antioxidants

One of the reasons why the Mediterranean Diet is so powerful is that it is naturally made of foods that are antioxidant rich. For example:

Food	Antioxidant
Red Wine	Resveratrol
Green Tea	Catechins
Pomegranates	Ellagitannins
Muscadine Grape	Resveratrol
Turmeric Curry Spice	Curcuminoids

Periodontitis–A heart disease risk factor

Your oral health can directly impact your heart health. Inflammation in your gums from periodontal disease increases the risk of cardiovascular disease. When your gums become infected, the bacteria in the affected periodontal tissue causes a generalized inflammatory response that increases the risk of heart attack and stroke.

Brushing and flossing your teeth regularly is key to preventing dental plaque buildup and reducing gingivitis, the beginnings of periodontal disease. Periodontal disease literally means infection and inflammation around the tooth, and it can affect one tooth or many. If you aren't brushing and flossing on a regular basis, small particles of food can get trapped between your teeth and gums and lead to infection and dental plaque formation. Your gums can become tender, red, even swollen, and can bleed following brushing. That inflammatory response, in which the body aggressively attacks the dental tissue and bone, results in receding gums and tooth loss. Even worse, chronic periodontal disease can lead to a state of chronic low-grade inflammation in the body. This can lead to a number of disease states, including heart disease.

There's more. A 2004 New York University and Centers for Disease Control (CDC) survey identified a link between periodontal disease and diabetes in almost three thousand patients. Dr. Sheila Strauss of NYU's Colleges of Dentistry and Nursing determined that 93% of participants with periodontal disease were considered to be high risk for diabetes, compared to just 63% of those without periodontal disease.

So make an appointment with a dentist, and see your dental hygienist for cleanings at least twice a year. In between cleanings, be sure to brush twice a day and floss every day.

Key Points

> Chronic inflammation increases the risk of many diseases, including heart disease and cancer.

- High sensitivity C-reactive protein (hs-CRP) is a biomarker of vascular inflammation.

- A landmark clinical trial (Jupiter) showed that in healthy people without high cholesterol but with elevated hs-CRP levels, a statin (rosuvastatin) significantly reduced the incidence of major cardiovascular events.

- Another important clinical trial (CANTOS) concluded that anti-inflammatory therapy for patients with a prior heart attack and elevated hs-CRP significantly lowered the rate of recurrent cardiovascular events.

- Two recent clinical trials showed that low dose colchicine, an anti-inflammatory agent used to treat gout, significantly lowered the risk of heart attack, stroke, and cardiovascular death in patients with acute and chronic coronary heart disease.

- The best way to prevent inflammation is to avoid the causes. Avoid the highly processed Western diet—instead follow a healthy diet like the Mediterranean diet that is rich in antioxidants (e.g., fruits and vegetables) and is anti-inflammatory (e.g., omega-3-rich fish).

- See your health care provider to properly treat pro-inflammatory disease states (e.g.,

arthritis, bronchitis, periodontitis, inflammatory bowel disease).

➤ Avoid inflammatory toxins like air pollution
and pesticide exposure.

CHAPTER **13**

High Blood Pressure –
The Silent Killer

Achieving Optimal Blood Pressure

Your blood pressure is the measure of the force of your blood against the artery wall. Systolic pressure is the pressure exerted on the artery wall as your heart beats; diastolic is the pressure exerted as your heart relaxes between beats. A normal blood pressure reading used to be less than 140/90 mmHg, with 120/80 mmHg as ideal.

Then along came the SPRINT trial. The SPRINT hypertension study was a randomized clinical trial that concluded that among patients at high risk for cardiovascular events, targeting a systolic blood pressure of less than 120 mmHg, as compared with less than 140 mmHg, resulted in lower rates of fatal and nonfatal major cardiovascular events and death from any cause. This landmark trial resulted in a marked change in hypertension guidelines and set normal blood pressure as less than 120/80 mmHg.

BLOOD PRESSURE CATEGORY	SYSTOLIC mm Hg (upper number)		DIASTOLIC mm Hg (lower number)
NORMAL	LESS THAN 120	and	LESS THAN 80
ELEVATED	120 – 129	and	LESS THAN 80
HIGH BLOOD PRESSURE (HYPERTENSION) STAGE 1	130 – 139	or	80 – 89
HIGH BLOOD PRESSURE (HYPERTENSION) STAGE 2	140 OR HIGHER	or	90 OR HIGHER
HYPERTENSIVE CRISIS (consult your doctor immediately)	HIGHER THAN 180	and/or	HIGHER THAN 120

Blood Pressure Measurement

The American Heart Association scientific statement on blood pressure measurement was modified following the SPRINT trial. In the office setting, many digital devices have been validated that allow accurate blood pressure measurement while reducing human errors associated with the auscultatory approach with a stethoscope. Fully automated digital devices capable of taking multiple readings, even without an observer being present, may provide a more accurate measurement of blood pressure than auscultation. Studies have shown substantial differences in blood pressure when measured outside versus in the office setting. Ambulatory blood pressure monitoring is considered the reference standard for out-of-office blood pressure assessment, with home blood pressure monitoring being an alternative when ambulatory blood pressure monitoring is not available or tolerated. In addition, high nighttime blood pressure on ambulatory blood pressure monitoring is associated with increased cardiovascular disease risk. Since digital blood pressure devices are now affordable and easy to use, many physicians now recommend that their patients monitor their blood pressure at home.

It is normal for your blood pressure to fluctuate during the day due to physical activity or stressful stimuli; however, it should return to normal as your body adjusts to whatever situation you're in. If it doesn't adjust, and it remains chronically elevated, then you will be diagnosed with hypertension. Hypertension is quite common, effecting more than fifty million Americans.

There are many causes of hypertension. The primary cause is aging. Blood vessels lose their elasticity as we age, and that causes a reduction in the ability to expand and contract. If you think of a balloon, this is how a young, healthy artery reacts when under pressure—it expands. But older arteries aren't flexible enough to expand, causing greater force against the artery wall. This can lead to a rise in systolic blood pressure, which may lead to a stroke, especially in the elderly.

Another common cause of hypertension is heredity. Some people are genetically more predisposed to having high blood pressure, which means life-style choices—like proper diet, exercise, and not smoking—are very important.

Hypertension that is caused by treatable conditions is called secondary hypertension, meaning it is the result of something else. You may be surprised to learn that one of the most common "treatable" conditions that cause hypertension is poor nutrition. Excessive salt intake leads to an elevated blood pressure. Too much alcohol or caffeine can also cause increased blood pressure. One question I always ask my patients is if they eat licorice. Licorice contains glycyrrhizin, a substance that can cause sodium retention and lead to hypertension. The Mediterranean diet, or DASH diet, are eating patterns that have been shown to lower blood pressure. Lack of exercise as well as chronic stress and anxiety contribute to high blood pressure. Lastly, obesity is an independent risk factor for the development and progression of hypertension, cardiovascular disease, and chronic kidney disease. Weight loss in overweight or obese patients can significantly lower blood pressure.

How common is secondary hypertension?

Because secondary is less common than primary hypertension, it is not always discovered. Testing for secondary hypertension can be expensive, so your healthcare provider will typically wait to begin testing until they strongly suspect secondary hypertension.

In addition, there are many different conditions or diseases that can cause secondary hypertension, including:

- **Kidney disease**: Poor blood flow to the kidney or injury to the kidney can trigger higher production of a hormone called renin. Renin leads to production of molecules like angiotensin that can raise blood pressure.
- **Adrenal disease**: Located on top of the kidneys, the adrenal glands produce and regulate hormones. When there is a problem with these glands, hormones in the body can become unbalanced and cause high blood pressure. Examples of adrenal conditions that can lead to high blood pressure include:
  - Pheochromocytoma—a tumor of the adrenal gland that overproduces epinephrine and norepinephrine—the fight-or-flight hormones
  - Primary aldosteronism—a condition where the body makes too much of the salt-retaining hormone aldosterone
  - Cushing's syndrome—a condition where there is too much of the hormone cortisol, a regulator of carbohydrate metabolism and blood pressure
- **Hyperparathyroidism**: the parathyroid glands (located in the neck), can overproduce hormones

that regulate calcium levels in the blood, and this condition may lead to high blood pressure.

- **Thyroid problems**: abnormal thyroid function (hyperthyroid or hypothyroid) may also lead to high blood pressure.
- **Coarctation (constriction or tightening) of the aorta**: This usually occurs beyond the blood vessels that branch off to your upper body and before the blood vessels that lead to your lower body. This can often lead to high blood pressure in your arms but low blood pressure in your legs and ankles.
- **Obstructive sleep apnea**: Caused by pauses in breathing during sleep due to collapsed passages in the upper airways. This condition can cause high blood pressure.

Side effects from certain medications can also contribute to secondary hypertension. Medications like:

- Hormonal contraceptives (birth control pills)
- Nonsteroidal anti-inflammatory agents (NSAIDs)
- Diet pills
- Stimulants
- Antidepressants
- Immune system suppressants
- Decongestants

Control Blood Pressure the Natural Way

- Limit sodium (<2,300 mg/day)
- Fruits and vegetables
- Pomegranate juice
- Daily exercise
- Smoking cessation
- Avoid trans fat
- Avoid alcohol excess
- Avoid caffeine excess
- Control stress
- Achieve ideal body weight
- Treat sleep apnea if present

Medications to control blood pressure

Before pharmaceutical therapy is started for blood pressure control, always exclude secondary causes of hypertension.

The three main types of medications to control blood pressure:

1. thiazide diuretic
2. calcium channel blocker (amlodipine)
3. angiotensin-converting-enzyme inhibitor or angiotensin receptor blocker.

These medications can be given alone or in combination to control blood pressure.

Remember, medications are never given in place of healthy lifestyle changes but rather in addition to them if needed to achieve optimal blood pressure.

Infrequently, blood pressure is not able to be controlled with therapeutic lifestyle intervention and medications. This is called resistant hypertension. If this occurs, a mineralocorticoid receptor blocker (spironolactone) is added to the medications listed above. If this type of medication is utilized, then electrolytes (esp. potassium) need to be monitored closely.

Key Points

> Hypertension is a major risk factor for cardiovascular disease.

> A normal blood pressure is <120/80 mmHg.

> Blood pressure should be controlled throughout life.

> Controlling blood pressure with a healthy lifestyle and blood pressure lowering medications (if needed) significantly lowers the risk of heart attack, stroke, vascular disease, and heart failure.

➤ Always exclude secondary causes of hypertension.

➤ A home digital blood pressure device is an easy and accurate way to monitor your blood pressure.

CHAPTER 14

Putting It All Together:
A Prescription to End
Heart Disease

We are at the dawn of a new era in our quest to prevent and eradicate atherosclerotic cardiovascular disease, the leading cause of death in America and worldwide. With healthy lifestyle choices and new medications that are now available, we are ready to attack and destroy this ruthless killer. It is now time to fight back! This is my prescription to end heart disease:

- Discuss a heart disease prevention plan with your personal physician.

- Maintain LDL cholesterol (50—70 mg/dl) throughout life with a healthy lifestyle and medications if needed.

- For those with existing coronary heart disease, follow a heart-healthy lifestyle and take statin medications and approved non-statin medications to achieve very low levels of LDL cholesterol (optimal <50 mg/dl).

- For those with early soft plaque identified on a vascular ultrasound or CT angiogram, institute lifestyle changes and medications to achieve a very low level of LDL cholesterol (<50mg/dl) to regress or eradicate the plaque, then return to maintaining LDL cholesterol 50–70 mg/dl with a healthy lifestyle and medications as needed.

- Maintain triglycerides <150 mg/dl (optimal <100 mg/dl) with a healthy lifestyle and medications as needed.

- Measure lipoprotein(a)—if elevated, maintain optimal levels <50 mg/dl with medical therapy if clinical trials, in progress, demonstrate a reduction in adverse cardiovascular events (e.g. heart attack and stroke).

- Measure the vascular inflammation biomarker hs-CRP (high-sensitivity C reactive protein) and maintain a level <2 mg/dl (optimal <1mg/dl) with lifestyle and medical therapy as needed.

- Measure fasting blood glucose, hemoglobin A1C, and fasting insulin levels, and maintain optimal levels with lifestyle intervention and medications as needed.

- Measure omega-3 and maintain optimal levels with omega-3-rich fish consumption and omega-3 medication as needed.

- Measure vitamin D and maintain level >30 mg/dl with lifestyle and medication as needed.

- Monitor blood pressure with a home digital BP device throughout life and maintain optimal BP <120/80 with a healthy lifestyle and medications as needed.

- Achieve high quality sleep (six to eight hours/ night). Get evaluated for sleep apnea if you snore or have daytime fatigue.

- Follow a Mediterranean diet.

- Exercise daily. Avoid prolonged sitting.

- Control stress with a healthy lifestyle and incorporate stress-reduction techniques as needed (relaxation response, yoga, meditation, mindfulness, prayer).

- Avoid smoking, vaping, and air pollution

Which Path to Take?

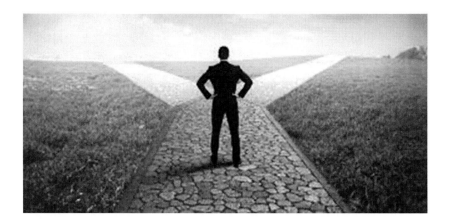

There are two paths to take in your battle against heart disease. One path is the **dead-end road**. Keep doing the same old thing: continue following the toxic, highly-processed American diet, remain physically inactive, feel "stressed out" most of the time, get poor quality sleep, accept an elevated LDL cholesterol and triglyceride level, have no idea what your lipoprotein(a) or hs-CRP levels are, and assume that your elevated blood pressure is "no big deal." The dead-end road leads to heart disease and numerous other diseases.

Then there is **progress road**. Following a healthy lifestyle, including optimal nutrition and regular exercise. Knowing what blood tests are important and making sure your blood levels are in the optimal range. Maintaining a normal blood pressure. Having a personal treating physician who takes the time to discuss a prevention strategy for defeating heart disease. Progress road leads to a long, happy, and heart-healthy life.

The decision is yours.
Wishing you all the best,
Michael Ozner, MD

Summary

> Atherosclerotic cardiovascular disease is the leading cause of death for men and women worldwide.

➢ What we are doing to halt this disease is not working. A new paradigm is needed to prevent atherosclerotic heart and vascular disease.

➢ The primary or root cause of this disease is an excessive number of cholesterol and triglyceride carrying atherogenic lipoproteins in the circulation; they enter the blood vessel wall, eventually leading to an atherosclerotic plaque. When these plaques rupture, a heart attack often occurs.

➢ Eliminate residual risk factors: poor nutrition, physical inactivity, high blood pressure, smoking, stress, insulin resistance and diabetes, lipoprotein(a), and inflammation.

➢ LDL cholesterol levels are a surrogate marker of the number of atherogenic lipoproteins.

➢ Lower is better—the lower the LDL cholesterol we can achieve with a healthy diet and medications (when needed), the lower the risk of heart attack and vascular disease.

➢ Earlier is better—the earlier in life we can achieve a lower LDL cholesterol, the better.

➢ Achieve optimal LDL cholesterol: 50 mg/dl to 70 mg/dl throughout life. In those with existing atherosclerotic plaques, achieve an LDL cholesterol less than 50 mg/dl to stabilize,

regress (shrink), and in some cases, eradicate plaques.

➤ Normal triglyceride level is less than 150
mg/dl, and optimal triglyceride level is less
than 100 mg/dl. Lowering triglyceride levels
lowers risk of heart attack.

➤ A landmark clinical trial demonstrated that
lowering elevated triglyceride levels, with a
highly purified omega-3 EPA ethyl ester, in
patients at high cardiovascular disease risk
who had optimal LDL cholesterol levels significantly lowered major adverse cardiovascular events (including heart attack and stroke).

➤ Genetics have paved the way for new medications that now allow us to safely achieve low
levels of LDL cholesterol, triglycerides, and
lipoprotein(a) that heretofore we were unable
to achieve.

➤ We are now at the dawn of a new era in our
quest to defeat cardiovascular disease.

Bibliography and Additional Reading

Gerber, Y., Rosen, L.J., Goldbourt, U., Benyamini, Y., Drory, Y. et al. Smoking status and long-term survival after first acute myocardial infarction: A population-based cohort study. *Journal of the Am. Col. of Cardiology.* Dec. 15, 2009;54(25):2382-2387.

Piano MR, Benowitz NL, FitzGerald GA, et al. Impact of smokeless tobacco products on cardiovascular disease. *Circulation* 2010; DOI:10.1161/CIR.0b013e3181f432c3. Available at: http://circ.ahajournals.org.

Bullen, C. Impact of tobacco smoking and smoking cessation on cardiovascular risk and disease. *Expert Review of Cardiovascular Therapy.* July 2008;6(6):883-895.

Erhardt L. Cigarette smoking: an undertreated risk factor for cardiovascular disease. *Atherosclerosis.* July 2009; 205(1):23-32.

Boffetta, P., Straif, K. Use of smokeless tobacco and risk of myocardial infarction and stroke: systemic review with meta-analysis. *BMJ.* Aug. 2009;339:b3060

Glick, M. and Greenburg, B.L. The potential role of dentists in identifying patients' risk of experience coronary artery disease events. *Journal of the American Dental Association.* Noc. 2005;136:1541-1546.

Jontell, M. and Glick, M. Oral health care professionals' identification of cardiovascular disease risk among patients in private dental offices in Sweden. *Journal of the American Dental Association.* Nov. 2009;140(11):1385-1391.

Strauss, S., et al. The dental office visit as a potential opportunity for diabetes screening: an analysis using NHANES 2003-2004 data. *Journal of Public Health Dentistry*. 70(2):156-162.

The American Dental Association
www.ada.org

Become an Ex-Smoker
www.becomeanex.org
Smokefree.gov

Keteyian, S. et al. American College of Cardiology's 58th Annual Scientific Session. Orlando, Florida.

Keteyian, S. et al. Exercise training in patients with heart failure. *Annals of Internal Medicine*. June 1996; 124(12):1051-1057.

Paffenbarger, R.S., Blair, S.N., Lee, I. A history of physical activity, cardiovascular health, and longevity: the scientific contributions of Jeremy N. Morris. *International Journal of Epidemiology*. 2001;30(5):1184-1192.

Madden, K.M., Lockhart, C., Cuff, D., et al. Short-term aerobic exercise reduces arterial stiffness in older adults with Type 2 diabetes, hypertension, and hypercholesterolemia. *Diabetes Care*. Aug. 2009;32(8):1531-1535.

Kelley, G.A., Med Kelley, K.A., Tran, Z.V. Aerobic exercise and resting blood pressure: a meta-analytic review of randomized, controlled trials. *Preventive Cardiology*. Spring 2001;4(2):73-80.

Morris, J. Vigorous exercise in leisure-time: protection against coronary artery disease. *The Lancet*. 316(8206):1207-1210.

Marieb, Elaine; Katja Hoehn (2007). *Human Anatomy & Physiology* (7th ed.). Pearson Benjamin Cummings. p. 317. ISBN 0805353879.

Chang, A.Y., et al. Cardiovascular risk factors and coronary atherosclerosis in retired National Football League players. *American Journal of Cardiology.* 2009;104(6):805-811.

Hunter, G.R. et al. Exercise training prevents regain of visceral fat for 1-year following weight loss. *Obesity.* April, 2010;18(4):690-695.

O'Connor, C.M., et al. Efficacy and safety of exercise training in patients with chronic heart failure. *Journal of the American Medical Association.* 2009;301(14):1439-1450.

Flynn, K.E. et al. Effects of exercise training on health status in patients with chronic heart failure: HF-ACTION randomized controlled trial. *JAMA.* 2009;301(14):1451-1459.

Lalande, S. et al. Effects of interval walking on physical fitness in middle-aged individuals. *Journal of Primary Care & Community.* July, 2010;1(2):104-110.

Roussel, M. et al. Influence of a walking program on the metabolic risk profile of obese postmenopausal women. *Menopause.* May/June 2009;16(3):566-575.

Sattelmair, J.R., Kurth, T., Buring, J.E., Lee, I.M. Physical activity and risk of stroke in women. *Stroke.* April, 2010;41(6):1243.

Bassett, D. R., Schneider, P.L., Huntington, G.E. Physical activity in an Old Order Amish community. *Med. Sci. Sports Exerc.* Jan. 2004;36(1):79-85.

Tudor-Locke, C. Steps to better cardiovascular health: how many steps does it take to achieve good health and how confident are we in this number? *Curr. Cardio Risk Rep.* 2010;4:271-276.

American College of Sports Medicine
www.acsm.org

American Heart Association
www.aha.org

Exercise is Medicine
www.exerciseismedicine.org

Nabi, H. et al. Effects of depressive symptoms and coronary heart disease and their interactive associations on mortality in middle-aged adults: the Whitehall II cohort study. *Heart*. Sept. 2010; doi:10.1136/hrt.2010.198507

Chris C. Streeter et al. Effects of Yoga Versus Walking on Mood, Anxiety, and Brain GABA Levels: A randomized controlled MRS study. *The Journal of Alternative and Complementary Medicine*, 2010; 16 (11): 1145 DOI: 10.1089/acm.2010.0007

Walters, K., Rait, G., Petersen, I., Williams, R., Nazareth, I. Panic disorder and risk of new onset coronary heart disease, acute myocardial infarction, and cardiac mortality: cohort study using the general practice research database. *European Heart Journal*. Oct. 2008;29(24);2981-2988. doi:10.1093/eurheartj/ehn477

Stewart, J.C., Rand, K.L., Muldoon, M.F., and Kamarck, T.W. A prospective evaluation of the directionality of the depression-inflammation relationship. *Brain, Behavior and Immunity*. Oct. 2009;23(7):936-944.

Martens, E.J., de Jonge, P., Na, B., Cohen, B.E., Lett, H., Whooley, M.A. Scared to death? Generalized anxiety disorder and cardiovascular events in patients with stable coronary heart disease. *Arch Gen Psychiatry*. 2010;67(7):750-758.

Kupper, N., Gidron, Y., Winter, J. and Denollet, J. Association between Type D personality, depression, and oxidative stress in patients with chronic heart failure. *Psychosomatic Med*. 2009;71:973-980.

Martens, E.J., Mols, F. Burg, M.M., Denollet, J. Type D personality and disease severity independently predict clinical events after myocardial infarction. *Journal Clinical Psychiatry.*2010;71(6):778-783.

Denollet, J., Schiffer, A., and Spek, V. A general propensity to psychological distress affects cardiovascular outcomes: Evidence from research on Type D (distressed) personality profile. *Circulation: Cardiovascular Quality and Outcomes.* 2010;3:546-557.

Ruberman, W., Weinblatt, A.B., Goldberg, J.D., Chaudhary, B.S. Psychosocial influences on mortality after myocardial infarction. *NEJM.* Aug. 1984;311:552-559.

Karelina, K., Norman, G.J., Zhang, N. Morris, Peng, H., DeVries, C. Social isolation alters neuroinflammatory response to stroke. *PNAS.* April, 2009;106(14):5895-5900.

Schneider, R., Nidich, S., Kotchen, J.M., Kotchen, T., Grim, C., Rainforth, M., King, C.G., Salerno, J. Effects of stress reduction on clinical events in African Americans with coronary heart disease: a randomized controlled trial. *Circulation.* 2009;120:S461.

Pullen, P.R. et al. Benefits of yoga for African American heart failure patients. *Med. & Sci in Sports & Exerc.* April 2010;42(4):651-657.

Kiecolt-Glaser, J.K. et al. Stress, inflammation, and yoga practice. *Psychosomatic Medicine.* 2010;72:1-9.

Kuntsevich, V., Bushell, W.C., Theise, N.D. Mechanisms of Yogic practices in health, aging and disease. *Mount Sinai Journal of Medicine.* Sept/Oct. 2010;77(5):559-569.

Uebelacker, L.A. et al. Hatha yoga for depression: critical review of the evidence for efficacy, plausible mechanisms of action, and directions for future research. *Journal of Psychiatric Practice.* Jan. 2010;16(1):22-33.

Naska, A., Oikonomou, E., Trichopoulou, A., Psaltopoulou, T., Trichopoulos, D. Siesta in healthy adults and coronary mortality in the general population. *Archives of Internal Medicine.* 2007;16793):296-301.

Sabanayagam, C., Shankar, A. Sleep duration and cardiovascular disease: results from the National Health Interview Survey. Aug. 2010;33(8).

Rafalson, L. et al. Short sleep duration is associated with the development of impaired fasting glucose: The Western New York Health Study. *Annals of Epidemiology.* Dec. 2010;20(12):883-889.

Donga, E. et al. A single night of partial sleep deprivation induces insulin resistance in multiple metabolic pathways in healthy subjects. *Journal of Clin. Endocrin & Metabol.* 2010;95(6):2963-2968.

Vlachopoulos, C., et al. Divergent effects of laughter and mental stress on arterial stiffness and central hemodynamics. *Psychosomatic Medicine.* March 2009; doi: 10.1097/PSY.0b013e318198dcd4

Sugawara, J., Tarumi, T., Tanaka, H. Effect of mirthful laughter on vascular function. *The American Journal of Cardiology.* Sept. 2010;106(6):856-859.

Miller, M., Fry, W. The effect of mirthful laughter on the human cardiovascular system. *Medical Hypotheses.* 2009;73:636-639.

American Association for Therapeutic Humor
www.aath.org

Laughter Yoga
www.laughteryoga.org

Hayman LL, Meininger, JC, et al. Primary prevention of cardiovascular disease in nursing practice: Focus on children and youth. *Circulation.* 2007;116:344-357.

Freiberg, MS, Pencina, MJ, D'Agostino RB, Lanier K, Wilson PW, Vasan RS. BMI vs. Waist circumference for identifying vascular risk. *Obesity*. 2008;16:463-469.

Rosito GA, Massaro JM, Hoffman U, Ruberg FL, Mahabadi AA, O'Donnell, CJ, Fox CS. Pericardial fat, visceral abdominal fat, cardiovascular disease risk factors, and vascular calcification in a community-based sample. *Circulation*. 2008;117:605-613.

Jalal DI, Ikizler, T. High fructose consumption is independently associated with high blood pressure. Renal Week 2009: American Society of Nephrology (ASN) 2009 Annual Meeting: Abstract TH-FC037. Presented October 29, 2009.

Daniel CR, Cross AJ, Koebnick C, Sinha R. Trends in red meat consumption in the USA. *Public Health Nutrition*. Published online Nox. 12, 2010.

Bernstein AM, Sun Q, Hu FB, Stampfer MJ, Manson JE, Willett WC. Major dietary protein sources and risk of coronary heart disease in women. *Circulation*. 2010;122:876-883.

Crowe, FL, Roddam, AW, Key, TJ et al. Fruit and vegetable intake and mortality from ischaemic heart disease: results from the European Prospective Investigation into Cancer and Nutrition (EPIC)-Heart study. *European Heart Journal*. Jan. 2011;32. Eur Heart J (2011) doi: 10.1093/eurheartj/ehq465

Lam TK, Cross AJ, Consonni D, Randi G, Bagnardi V, Bertazzi PB, Caporaso NE, Sinha R, Subar AF, Landi MT. Intakes of red meat, processed meat and meat mutagens increase lung cancer risk. *Cancer Research*. 2009;69:932.

Wu X, Lin J, et al. University of Texas M. D. Anderson Cancer Center (2010, April 20). Meat, especially if it's well done, may increase risk of bladder cancer. *ScienceDaily*.

Retrieved January 22, 2011, from http://www.science-daily.com /releases/2010/04/100419150827.htm

Fung TT, Rexrode KM, Mantzoros CS, Manson JE, Willett WC, Hu FB. Mediterranean diet and incidence of and mortality from coronary heart disease and stroke in women. *Circulation*. 2009;119:1093-1100.

Yusuf S, Hawken S, Ounpuu S, et al., INTER-HEART study investigators. Effect of potentially modifiable risk factors associated with myocardial infarction in 52 countries (the INTER-HEART study):case-control study. *The Lancet* 2004;364:937-952.

O'Keefe, T, Bybee, K, Lavie, C. Alcohol and cardiovascular health: The razor-sharp double-edge sword. *Journal of the American College of Cardiology*. 2007;50(11):1009-1014.

Micha R, Wallace SK, Mozaffarian D. Red and processed meat consumption and risk of incident coronary heart disease, stroke and diabetes mellitus. *Circulation*. 2010;121:2271-2283.

Puangsombat K, Smith JS. Inhibition of heterocyclic amine formation in beef patties by ethanolic extracts of rosemary. *Journal of Food Science*. Mar 2010;75(2):T40-T47.

Smith, J.S., Ameri, F., Gadgil, P. Effect of marinades on the formation of heterocyclic amines in grilled beef steaks. Journal of Food Science. April 2008;73(6):T100-T105.

Steck SE, Hebert JR. GST polymorphism and excretion of heterocyclic aromatic amine and isothiocyanate metabolites after Brassica consumption. *Environmental and Molecular Mutagenesis*. April 2009;50(3):238-246.

New York City Department of Health and Mental Hygiene. Statement on Trans Fats. http://www.nyc.gov/html/doh/html/cardio/cardio-transfat.shtml Accessed 1/21/11.

State of California statement on banning of trans fats. http://cchealth.org/groups/eh/retail_food/pdf/ab97_transfat_ban_guidelines.pdf Accessed 1/21/11.

City of Boston Public Health Commission statement of banning trans fats. http://www.bphc.org/programs/cib/chronicdisease/heal/transfat/Pages/Home.aspx Accessed 1/21/11.

Mayo Clinic Health Information. Artificial Sweeteners: Understanding these and other sugar substitutes. http://www.mayoclinic.com/health/artificial-sweeteners/MY00073 Accessed 1/21/11.

Degirolamo C, Shelness GS, Rudel LL. LDL cholesteryl oleate as a predictor for atherosclerosis: evidence from human and animal studies on dietary fat. *The Journal of Lipid Research.* April 2009;50:S434-S439.

Ostman E, Granfeldt Y, Persson L, Bjorck I. Vinegar supplementation lowers glucose and insulin responses and increases satiety after a bread meal in healthy subjects. *Euro Journal Clin Nutr.* 2005;59:983-988.

Konstantinidou V, Covas MI, et al. In vivo nutrigenomic effects of virgin olive oil polyphenols within the frame of the Mediterranean diet: a randomized controlled trial. *The FASEB Journal.* July 2010;24(7):2546-2557.

Sun Q, Spiegelman D, van Dam RM, Holmes, MD, Malik VS, Willett WC, Hu FB. White rice, brown rice, and risk of Type 2 diabetes in U.S. men and women. *Archives of Internal Medicine.* 2010;170(11):961-969.

Sakata Y, Zhuang H, Kwansa H, Koehler RC, Dore S. Resveratrol protects against experimental stroke: putative neuroprotective role of heme oxygenase 1. *Experimental Neurology.* July 2010;224(1):325-329.

Arab L, Liu W, Elashoff D. Both black and green tea consumption associated with reduced risk of stroke. *The FASEB Journal.* April 2009;23 Meeting Abstract Supplement:345.5

Wang, Z., Zhou, B., Wang, Y., Gong, Q., Wang, Q., Yan, J., Gao, W., Wang, L. Black and green tea consumption and the risk of coronary artery disease: a meta-analysis. Jan. 2011;93(1).

Nilsson M, Holst J, Bjorck, I. Metabolic effects of amino acid mixtures and whey protein in healthy subjects: studies using glucose-equivalent drinks. *American Journal of Clinical Nutrition.* 2007;85:996-1004.

O'Keefe, J., Gheewala, N., O'Keefe, J. Dietary strategies for improving post-prandial glucose, lipids, inflammation, and cardiovascular health. *American Journal of Cardiology.* 2008;51(3):249-255.

Djousse L, Hopkins PN, North KE, Pankow JS, Arnett DK, Ellison RC. Chocolate consumption is inversely associated with prevalent coronary heart disease: The National Heart, Lung, and Blood Institute Family Heart Study. *Clinical Nutrition.* Article in press at time of publishing.

Crawford P. Effectiveness of cinnamon for lowering hemoglobin A1C in patients with Type 2 diabetes: a randomized, controlled trial. *The Journal of the American Board of Family Medicine.* 2009;22(5):507-512.

Ried K, Sullivan T, Fakler P, Frank OR, Stocks NP. Does chocolate reduce blood pressure? A meta-analysis. *BMC Medicine.* 2010;8(39)

Dai J, Lampert R, Wilson PW, Goldberg J, Ziegler TR, Vaccarino V. Mediterranean dietary pattern is associated with improved cardiac autonomic function among middle-aged men. *Circulation: Cardiovascular Quality and Outcomes.* June 2010.

Trichopoulou A, Bamia C, Lagiou P, Trichopoulos D. Conformity to traditional Mediterranean diet and breask cancer risk in the Greek EPIC (European Prospective Investigation into Cancer and Nutrition) cohort. *American Journal of Clinical Nutrition.* Sept 2010;92(3): 620-625.

Scarmeas N, Stern Y, Mayeux R, Manly JJ, Schupf N, Luchsinger JA. Mediterranean diet and mild cognitive impairment. *Archives of Neurology.* 2009;66(2):216-225.

Scarmeas N, Luchsinger JA, Schupf N, Brickman AM, Cosentino S, Tang MX, Stern Y. Physical activity, diet and risk of Alzheimer disease. *JAMA.* 2009;302(6):627-637.

Sanchez-Villegas A, Delgado-Rodriguez M et al. Association of the Mediterranean dietary pattern with the incidence of depression: The Seguimento Universidad de Navarra cohort. *Archives of General Psychiatry.* 2009; 66(10):1090-1098

National Cholesterol Education Program. http://www.nhlbi. nih.gov/about/ncep/ Accessed 1/21/11.

Lovely RS, Kazmierczak SC, Massaro JM, D'Agostino Sr. RB, O'Donnell CJ, and Farrell DH. γ′ Fibrinogen: Evaluation of a New Assay for Study of Associations with Cardiovascular Disease. *Clin Chem.* 2010;56:781-788.

Nissen, SE, Nicholls, SJ, et al. Effects of very high-intensity statin therapy on regression of coronary atherosclerosis. *JAMA.* 2006;295(13):1556-1565.

Karlsson K, Ahlborg B, Dalman C, Hemmingsson T. Association between erythrocyte sedimentation rate and IQ in Swedish males aged 18-20. *Brain, Behavior and Immunity.* Aug 2010;24(6):868-873.

Miller KA, Siscovick DS, Sheppard L, Shepherd K, Sullivan JH, Anderson GL, Kaufman JD. Long-term exposure to air pollution and incidence of cardiovascular events in women. *New England Journal of Medicine.* Feb 2007;356:447-458.

Villareal-Calderon R, Palacios-Moreno J, Parker K, Calderon-Garciduenas L. Gene inflammatory expression profiling in right versus left ventricles in young urbanites: what is the long-term impact of myocardial inflammation in the setting of air pollution? *The FASEB Journal.* April 2010;24 Meeting Abstract Supplement. 1029.1

Silverman RA, Ito K, Freese J, Kaufman BJ, De Claro D, Braun J, Prezant DJ. Association of ambient fine particles with out-of-hospital cardiac arrests in New York City. *American Journal of Epidemiology.* Aug. 2010. doi: 10.1093/aje/kwq217 http://aje.oxfordjournals.org/content/early/2010/08/20/aje.kwq217.full.pdf+html Accessed 1/21/11.

Bauer M, Moebus S, Mohlenkamp S, Dragano N, Nonnemacher M, Fuchsluger M, Kessler C, Jakobs H, Memmesheimer M, Erbel R, Jockel KH, Hoffman B. Urban particulate matter air pollution is associated with subclinical atherosclerosis: results from the HNR (Heinz Nixdorf Recall) study. *Journal of the American College of Cardiology.* Nov. 2010;56(23):1803-1808.

Pearson, JF, Bachireddy C, Shyamprasad S, Godlfine AB, Brownstein JS. Association between fine particulate matter and diabetes prevalence in the U.S. *Diabetes Care.* Oct 2010;33(10):2196-2201.

Araujo JA, Barajas B, Kleinman M, Wang X, Bennett BJ, Gong KW, Navab M, Harkema J, Sioutas C, Lusis AJ, Nel AE. Ambient particulate pollutants in the ultrafine range promote early atherosclerosis and system oxidative stress. *Circulation Research.* 2008;102:589-596.

Viera L, Chen K, Nel A, Lloret MG. The impact of air pollutants as an adjuvant for allergic sensitization and asthma. *Current Allergy and Asthma Reports.* 2009;9(4):327-333.

Ghamin H, Sia CL, Abuaysheh S, Korzeniewski K, Patnaik P, Marumganti A, Chaudhuri A, Dandone P. An anti-inflammatory and reactive oxygen species suppressive effects of an extract of *Polygonum Cuspidatum* containing resveratrol. *Journal of Clinical Endocrinology & Metabolism.* 2010;95(9):E1-E8.

Gorelik S, Ligumsky M, Koehn R, Kanner J. A novel function of red wine polyphenols in humans: prevention of absorption of cytotoxic lipid peroxidation products. *The FASEB Journal.* Jan. 2008;22(1):41-46.

Li L, Seeram NP. Maple syrup phytochemicals include lignans, coumarins, a stilbene, and other previously unreported antioxidant phenolic compounds. Journal of Agriculture and Food Chemistry. 2010;58(22):11673-11679.

Ridker P, Danielson E, Fonseca F, Genest J, et al. Reduction in C-reactive protein and LDL cholesterol and cardiovascular event rates after initiation of rosuvastatin: a prospective study of the JUPITER trial. *The Lancet.* 2009;373(9670):1175-1182.

Harvard Medical School Publication on Glycemic Index. http://www.health.harvard.edu/newsweek/Glycemic_index_and_glycemic_load_for_100_foods.htm Accessed 1/21/11.

Murphy P, Fitchett G. Belief in a concerned god predicts response to treatment for adults with clinical depression. *Journal of Clinical Psychology.* Sept 2009;65(9):1000-1008.

Anderson JL, May HT, Horne BD, Bair TL, Hall NL, Carlquist JF, Lappe DL, Muhlestein JB. Relation of vitamin D deficiency to cardiovascular risk factors, disease status, and incident events in a general healthcare population. *American Journal of Cardiology* 2010 Oct 1;106(7):963-8.

Don Y, Stallmann-Jorgensen S, Pollock NK, Harris RA, Keeton D, Huang Y, Li K, Bassali R, Guo D, Thomas J, Pierce GL, White J, Holick MF, Zhu H. A 16-week randomized clinical trial of 2000 International Units daily vitamin D3 supplementation in Black youth: 25-hydroxyvitamin D, adiposity, and arterial stiffness. *Journal of Clinical Endocrinology & Metabolism.* 2010;95(10):4584-4591.

Bolland MJ, Avenell A, Baron JA, Grey A, MacLennan GA, Gamble GD, Reid IR. Effect of calcium supplements on a risk of myocardial infarction and cardiovascular events: meta-analysis. *British Medical Journal.* 2010;341:c3691.

Makhija N, Sendasgupta C, Kiran U, Lakshmy R, Hote MP, Chourhary SK, Airan B, Abraham R. The role of oral coenzyme Q10 in patients undergoing coronary artery bypass graft surgery. *Cardiothoracic and Vascular Anesthesia.* Dec 2008;22(6):832-839.

Schaars CF, Stalenhoef AF. Effects ubiquinone (coenzyme Q10) on myopathy in statin users. *Current Opinion in Lipidology.* Dec. 2008;19(6):553-557.

Leon H, Shibata MC, Sivakumaran S, Dorgan M, Chatterley T, Tsuyuki RT. Effect of fish oil on arrhythmias and mortality: systematic review. *The British Medical Journal.* 2008;337:a2931.

Barbosa VM, Miles EA, Calhau C, Lafuente E, Calder PC. Effects of fish oil containing lipid emulsion on plasma phospholipids fatty acids, inflammatory markers, and clinical outcomes in septic patients: a randomized, controlled clinical trial. *Critical Care.* 2010:14:R5.

Shargorodsky M, Debby O, Matas Z, Zimlichman R. Effect of long-term treatment with antioxidants (vitamin C, vitamin E, coenzyme Q10 and selenium) on arterial compliance, humoral factors, and inflammatory markers in patients with multiple cardiovascular risk factors. *Nutrition & Metabolism.* 2010;7:55.

Selected Recipes and Menu Plans from *The Complete Mediterranean Diet*

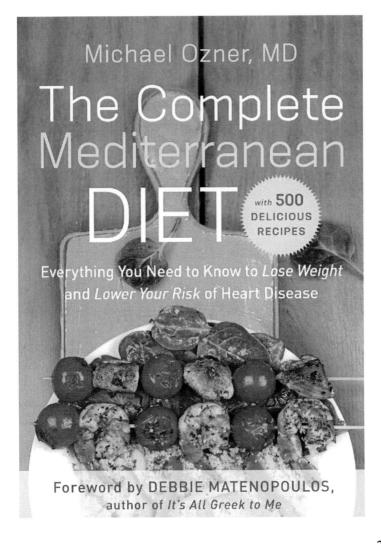

In order to defeat heart disease and have a long and healthy life, it is essential that you eat foods that are nutritious, delicious, and promote cardiovascular health. The best way to ensure healthy nutrition is to prepare the meals yourself. Preparing heathy and nutritious meals can be fun. In addition, it can be better for your health and more cost effective than eating restaurant or fast food. Lastly, the Mediterranean diet has been shown to be one of the most effective diets to lose weight and gain long-term health. To get you started, I have included a seven-day menu plan along with appetizers, main courses, side dishes, soups, and salads.

Many more recipes like these and an extended 14-day menu plan are found in *The Complete Mediterranean Diet*.

Seven-Day Menu Plan

Day 1

Breakfast

4 ounces vegetable or fruit juice

1 slice whole wheat toast drizzled with extra-virgin olive oil or 1 teaspoon vegetable spread (trans fat-free canola/olive oil spread)

1 teaspoon jam

½ cup plain low-fat yogurt (sweetened with non-caloric sweetener if desired)

½ cup blueberries or strawberries

8 ounces water

Coffee or tea (soy or non-fat milk, trans fat-free coffee creamer, and non-caloric sweetener if desired)

- Approx. 239 calories

Optional Midmorning Snack

10–20 almonds or walnuts

8 ounces water or non-caloric beverage

Lunch

Chickpea Pita Pocket

1 medium apple, sliced and drizzled with honey

8 ounces water or non-caloric beverage

- Approx. 319 ounces

Optional Midday Snack

10–20 almonds or walnuts

8 ounces water or non-caloric beverage

Dinner

1 jumbo clove Roasted Garlic

½ (6-inch) whole wheat pita loaf, split open, lightly sprayed with extra-virgin olive oil and herb seasonings of choice, and toasted in the microwave or oven until crispy

Goat Cheese Stuffed Tomato

Linguine and Mixed Seafood

Fresh vegetable of choice (flavor with a drizzle of extra-virgin olive oil or vegetable spread as desired)

Drunken Apricots

8 ounces of water

1 or 2 (5-ounce) glasses of red wine or purple grape juice

Coffee or tea (soy or non-fat milk, trans fat-free coffee creamer, and non-caloric sweetener if desired)

- Approx. 761 calories

Optional Evening Snack

1 apple or orange

8 ounces of water

Day 2

Breakfast

4 ounces vegetable or fruit juice

½ cup egg whites with diced onions, tomato, and green bell peppers cooked into an omelet

1 slice whole wheat toast drizzled with extra-virgin olive oil or 1 teaspoon vegetable spread (trans fat-free canola/olive oil spread)

1 teaspoon fruit jam

½ banana

8 ounces water

Coffee or tea (soy or non-fat milk, trans fat-free coffee creamer, and non-caloric sweetener if desired)

- Approx. 230 calories

Optional Midmorning Snack

10–20 almonds or walnuts

8 ounces water or non-caloric beverage

Lunch

Greek Olive and Feta Cheese Pasta Salad with slice of cantaloupe

8 ounces water or non-caloric beverage

- Approx. 354 calories

Optional Midday Snack

10–20 almonds or walnuts

8 ounces water or non-caloric beverage

Dinner

1 jumbo clove Roasted Garlic

½ (6-inch) whole wheat pita loaf, split open, lightly sprayed with extra-virgin olive oil and herb seasonings of choice, and toasted until crispy in the oven or microwave.

6–8 marinated assorted olives

Grilled Citrus Salmon with Garlic Greens

Grilled Eggplant

Strawberries and Balsamic Syrup

8 ounces water

1 or 2 (5-ounce) glasses of red wine or purple grape juice

Coffee or tea (soy or non-fat milk, trans fat-free coffee creamer, and non-caloric sweetener if desired)

• Approx. 653 calories

Optional Evening Snack

1 apple or 1 cup of bite-size pieces of watermelon, rind removed

8 ounces of water

Day 3

Breakfast

4 ounces vegetable or fruit juice

½ cup egg whites with diced onions, tomato, and spinach cooked into an omelet

1 slice whole wheat toast drizzled with extra-virgin olive oil or 1 teaspoon vegetable spread (trans fat-free canola/olive oil spread)

1 teaspoon fruit jam

1 medium fresh peach or 1 large plum

8 ounces water

Coffee or tea (soy or non-fat milk, trans fat-free coffee creamer, and non-caloric sweetener if desired)

• Approx. 230 calories

Optional Midmorning Snack

10–20 almonds or walnuts

8 ounces water or non-caloric beverage

Lunch

Italian Minestrone with Pesto

1 slice whole grain crusty bread, drizzled with extra-virgin olive oil

½ cup fresh raspberries

½ cup plain low-fat yogurt

8 ounces water or non-caloric beverage

• Approx. 390 calories

Optional Midday Snack

1 apple

8 ounces water or non-caloric beverage

Dinner

Simple Spanish Salad

1 jumbo clove of Roasted Garlic

½ (6-inch) whole wheat pita loaf, split open, lightly sprayed with extra-virgin olive oil and herb seasonings of choice, and toasted until crispy in the oven or microwave

1 slice of soft goat cheese

6–8 marinated mixed olives

Fresh vegetable of choice (flavor with a drizzle of extra-virgin olive oil or vegetable spread if desired)

Chicken Piccata

Honeydew Sorbet

8 ounces of water

1 or 2 (5-ounce) glasses of red wine or purple grape juice

Coffee or tea (soy or non-fat milk, trans fat-free coffee creamer, and non-caloric sweetener if desired)

- Approx. 725 calories

Optional Evening Snack

2 Meringue Cookies

Green tea or 8 ounces of water

Day 4

Breakfast

4 ounces of vegetable or fruit juice

2 slices of whole wheat toast

2 tablespoons of fresh chunky peanut butter

2 tablespoons honey

½ ruby red grapefruit, sweetened with non-caloric sweetener if desired

8 ounces water

Coffee or tea (soy or non-fat milk, trans fat-free coffee creamer, and non-caloric sweetener if desired)

- Approx. 385 calories

Optional Midmorning Snack

10-20 almonds or walnuts

8 ounces of water or non-caloric beverage

Lunch

Light Caesar Salad

1 slice Pizza Margherita

10-20 seedless grapes

8 ounces water or non-caloric beverage

• Approx. 302 calories

Optional Midday Snack

1 apple

8 ounces of water or non-caloric beverage

Dinner

Chilly Tomato Soup

Fennel Salad

Spicy Whole Wheat Capellini with Fresh Garlic

Fresh vegetable of your choice (flavor with a drizzle of extra-virgin olive oil or vegetable spread if desired)

½ (6-inch) whole wheat pita loaf, split open, lightly sprayed with extra-virgin olive oil and herb seasonings of choice, and toasted until crispy in the oven or microwave

Spicy Plum Compote

8 ounces of water

1 or 2 (5-ounce) glasses of red wine or purple grape juice

Coffee or tea (soy or non-fat milk, trans fat-free coffee creamer, and non-caloric sweetener if desired)

- Approx. 786 calories

Optional Evening Snack

1 apple or orange

8 ounces of water

Day 5

Breakfast

4 ounces of vegetable or fruit juice

1 slice whole wheat toast drizzled with extra-virgin olive oil or 1 teaspoon vegetable spread (trans fat-free canola/olive oil spread)

1 teaspoon fruit jam

½ cup plain low-fat yogurt, sweetened with non-caloric if desired

½ cup blueberries or strawberries (fresh or frozen, defrosted)

8 ounces water

Coffee or tea (soy or non-fat milk, trans fat-free coffee creamer, and non-caloric sweetener if desired)

- Approx. 289 calories

Optional Midmorning Snack

10-20 almonds or walnuts

8 ounces water or non-caloric beverage

Lunch

Hearty Bean Soup

1 slice whole grain bread drizzled with extra-virgin olive oil or 1 teaspoon vegetable spread (trans fat-free canola/olive oil spread)

3 fresh apricots

8 ounces water or non-caloric beverage

Optional Midday Snack

1 apple

8 ounces water or non-caloric beverage

Dinner

Fettuccine with Smoked Salmon and Basil Pesto

4 tablespoons hummus

½ (6-inch) whole wheat pita loaf, split open, lightly sprayed with extra-virgin olive oil and herb seasonings of choice, and toasted until crispy in the oven

4 tomato wedges topped with slivers of red onion, freshly grated mozzarella cheese, chopped fresh cilantro, and drizzled with aged balsamic vinegar and 1 teaspoon extra-virgin olive oil

Peach Marsala Compote

8 ounces of water

1 or 2 (5-ounce) glasses of red wine or purple grape juice

Coffee or tea (soy or non-fat milk, trans fat-free coffee creamer, and non-caloric sweetener if desired)

- Approx. 774 calories

Optional Evening Snack

2 Meringue Cookies

Green tea or 8 ounces water

Day 6

Breakfast

4 ounces of vegetable or fruit juice

½ cup dry oatmeal, cooked and sweetened with non-caloric sweetener if desired

1 tablespoon seedless black raisins

1 medium orange, sliced

8 ounces water

Coffee or tea (soy or non-fat milk, trans fat-free coffee creamer, and non-caloric sweetener if desired)

- Approx. 292 calories

Optional Midmorning Snack

10–20 almonds or walnuts

8 ounces water or non-caloric beverage

Lunch

Veggie Wrap

Roasted Peppers

6–8 marinated mixed olives

1 medium fresh pear, peach, or apple

8 ounces water or non-caloric beverage

• Approx. 601 calories

Optional Midday Snack

1 apple

8 ounces water or non-caloric beverage

Dinner

1 jumbo clove Roasted Garlic

½ (6-inch) whole wheat pita loaf, split open, lightly sprayed with extra-virgin olive oil and herb seasonings of choice, and toasted until crispy in the oven or microwave

Mediterranean Mixed Greens

Baked Tilapia

Classic Spinach and Pine Nuts

Strawberries Amaretto

8 ounces of water

1 or 2 (5-ounce) glasses of red wine or purple grape juice

Coffee or tea (soy or non-fat milk, trans fat-free coffee creamer, and non-caloric sweetener if desired)

- Approx. 597 calories

Optional Evening Snack

2 Meringue Cookies

Green tea or 8 ounces of water

Day 7

Breakfast

4 ounces of vegetable or fruit juice

½ cup egg whites with diced onion, tomato, and green bell peppers cooked into an omelet

1 slice whole wheat toast drizzled with extra-virgin olive oil or 1 teaspoon vegetable spread (trans fat-free canola/olive oil spread)

1 teaspoon fruit jam

1 purple plum

8 ounces water

Coffee or tea (soy or non-fat milk, trans fat-free coffee creamer, and non-caloric sweetener if desired)

- Approx. 230 calories

Optional Midmorning Snack

10–20 walnuts or almonds

8 ounces water or non-caloric beverage

Lunch

Eggplant Soup

1 slice whole grain crusty bread, drizzled with extra-virgin olive oil and herb seasonings of choice

1 large kiwi fruit, sliced

½ cup fresh strawberries, sliced

8 ounces water or non-caloric beverage

Approx. 420 calories

Optional Midday Snack

1 apple

8 ounces water or non-caloric beverage

Dinner

1 slice whole grain bread, drizzled with extra-virgin olive oil and herb seasonings of choice

6–8 marinated assorted olives

Broccoli with Fresh Garlic

Fettuccine with Sundried Tomatoes and Goat Cheese

Fresh Fruit Kabobs and Cinnamon Honey Dip

8 ounces of water

1 or 2 (5-ounce) glasses of red wine or purple grape juice

Coffee or tea (soy or non-fat milk, trans fat-free coffee creamer, and non-caloric sweetener if desired)

- Approx. 1050 calories

Optional Evening Snack

1 apple or orange

8 ounces of water

How do I prepare healthy and delicious Mediterranean meals? Not to worry, listed below are some of my favorite recipes–from appetizers to desserts, and everything in between.

Appetizers

Roasted Garlic

(makes 4–5 servings)

Preheat oven to 400 degrees

1 elephant jumbo garlic head

Extra-virgin olive oil to drizzle

Dry seasonings of choice (optional)

Holding entire head of garlic, cut off the top lead points of each clove to expose a small portion of the clove. Keep the remainder of leaves intact around the body of the garlic head. Place trimmed garlic head in a tight-fitting oven-safe bowl, trimmed side up. Drizzle a small amount of olive oil over the top of the head and down around the sides. Sprinkle with your favorite seasoning (optional). Place garlic on middle rack of oven and bake at 400 degrees for 20–30 minutes, or until cloves are soft and a light golden brown. Remove from oven and spread roasted garlic cloves on crusty bread, or add to vegetables, omelets, or pasta.

Approx. 59 calories per serving

Goat Cheese Stuffed Tomatoes

(makes 2 servings)

6–8 leaves fresh arugula

2 medium ripe tomatoes

3 ounces goat cheese

Salt and pepper to taste

Balsamic vinegar

Extra-virgin olive oil

Red onion, very thinly sliced

Fresh chopped parsley

Cut tops (about ¼ inch) off the tomatoes. With a paring knife, core out the center of the tomatoes, about ½ inch deep. Fill tomatoes with crumbled goat cheese, add salt and pepper to taste. Place 3–4 arugula leaves in the center of each salad plate, then place the tomatoes on the arugula. Drizzle with balsamic vinegar and extra-virgin olive oil. Garnish with red onion slices and chopped parsley.

Approx. 142 calories per serving

Salads

Simple Spanish Salad

(makes 6 servings)

1 bag (2 bunches) romaine lettuce, cleaned, trimmed, and torn into bite-size pieces

3 medium ripe tomatoes cut into ¼ inch wedges

1 large sweet onion, thinly sliced

1 green bell pepper, seeded and thinly sliced

1 red bell pepper, seeded and thinly sliced

¼ cup chopped and pitted marinated black olives

¼ cup chopped and pitted marinated green olives

¼ cup extra-virgin olive oil

3 tablespoons balsamic vinegar

Salt and freshly ground pepper to taste

Place a bed of romaine lettuce on six chilled salad plates. Arrange tomatoes, onions, peppers, and olives on top of the lettuce on each plate. Mix olive oil and vinegar together, drizzle over salad. Add salt and pepper if desired and serve.

Approx. 107 calories per serving

Light Caesar Salad

(makes 6 servings)

1–2 bunches romaine lettuce, cleaned, trimmed and torn into bite size pieces

½ cup non-fat plain yogurt

2 teaspoons lemon juice

2 ½ teaspoons balsamic vinegar

1 teaspoon Worcestershire sauce

2 cloves freshly minced garlic

½ teaspoon anchovy paste

½ cup grated Parmesan cheese

10 small pitted black olives, chopped

Place lettuce in large salad bowl. In a blender add yogurt, lemon juice, vinegar, Worcestershire sauce, garlic, anchovy paste, and ¼ cup Parmesan cheese and blend until smooth. Pour mixture over lettuce and toss. Garnish with remaining cheese and olives.

Approx. 49 calories

Fennel Salad

(makes 4-6 servings)

1 large clove garlic, halved

1 large fennel bulb, thinly sliced

½ English cucumber, thinly sliced

1 tablespoon minced fresh chives

8 large radishes, thinly sliced

3 tablespoons extra-virgin olive oil

2 ½ tablespoons freshly squeezed lemon juice

Salt and freshly ground pepper to taste

Marinated mixed olives (optional)

Rub the inside of a large bowl with garlic. Add fennel, cucumber, chive, and radishes. In a separate bowl whisk together olive oil, fresh lemon juice, and salt and pepper to taste. Pour olive oil mixture over salad and toss to mix. Garnish with marinated olives if desired.

Approx. 76 calories per serving

Mediterranean Mixed Greens
(makes 4–6 servings)

6 cups assorted fresh mixed greens (such as arugula, radicchio, baby spinach, watercress, and romaine)

1 small red onion, thinly sliced and separated into rings

20 firm cherry tomatoes, halved

¼ chopped walnuts

¼ dried cranberries

For dressing:
2 tablespoons balsamic vinegar

4 tablespoons extra-virgin olive oil

1 tablespoon water

½ teaspoon crushed dried oregano

2 cloves garlic, finely minced

Crumbled feta cheese (optional)

Freshly ground pepper to taste

In a large salad bowl, combine greens, onions, tomatoes, walnuts, and cranberries. Gently toss.

Dressing:
Combine vinegar, oil, water, oregano, and garlic; shake well. Pour dressing over salad and toss lightly to coat. Garnish with feta cheese, if desired, and fresh pepper.

Approx. 140 calories per serving

Soups

Italian Minestrone Soup with Pesto
(makes 6–8 servings)

1 cup dried cannellini beans

4 cups low-sodium, fat-free chicken broth

4 cups water

2 medium white potatoes, peeled and diced

2 ounces dry ditalini pasta

2 large carrots, chopped

3 stalks celery, chopped

½ cup chopped white onion

2 cloves garlic, minced

1 cup tomato juice

3 plum tomatoes, chopped

1 large zucchini, chopped

Freshly shredded Parmesan cheese for garnish (optional)

For pesto:

1 cup fresh basil leaves

1 teaspoon crumbled dried basil leaves

4 cloves garlic, finely minced

3 tablespoons extra-virgin olive oil

½ cup grated Parmesan cheese

Salt and freshly ground pepper to taste

Rinse cannellini beans and place in a large covered pot. Add chicken broth and water and bring to a boil. Uncover pot, reduce heat, and simmer until beans are tender; roughly one hour. Add potatoes, pasta, carrots, celery, onion, garlic, and tomato juice. Return mixture to boil, and then reduce heat and simmer uncovered for 10 minutes. Add tomatoes and zucchini, and simmer until all are tender. Process pesto ingredients in a food processor or blender until finely chopped. Remove soup from heat and stir in pesto mixture, and serve garnished with Parmesan cheese if desired.

Without pesto: Approx. 182 calories per serving
With pesto: Approx. 254 calories per serving

Chilly Tomato Soup
(makes 4 servings)

10 medium-ripe tomatoes
½ tablespoon extra-virgin olive oil
4-5 cloves garlic, minced
2 tablespoons chopped onions
2 cups low-sodium, fat-free chicken broth
2 teaspoons low-calorie baking sweetener
½ teaspoon chopped fresh basil
Salt and fresh ground pepper to taste
8 scallions, chopped (optional)
2 cucumbers, diced (optional)
1 large zucchini, diced (optional)

In a large pot of boiling water, dip tomatoes for 30 seconds, then immediately place tomatoes in cold water. Allow to sit until they can be handled. Skin tomatoes with a paring knife, cut in half crosswise, and remove seeds. Core and then cut into quarter pieces. In a blender or food processor, process tomatoes until pureed. In a skillet, heat olive oil and sauté garlic and onions until tender. Remove from heat. In a large bowl, combine pureed tomatoes, sautéed onion mixture, chicken broth, sweetener, basil, and salt and pepper, stirring to mix ingredients together. Refrigerate soup for 4–6 hours until well chilled. Garnish with scallions, cucumbers, and zucchini if desired.

Approx. 161 calories per serving

Eggplant Soup

(makes 4–6 servings)

2 tablespoons extra-virgin olive oil
2 cloves fresh garlic, minced
½ medium onion, thinly sliced and separated into rings
1 medium eggplant, peeled and cut into ½ inch cubes
½ teaspoon oregano
¼ teaspoon thyme
4 cups low-sodium, fat-free chicken broth
½ cup dry sherry
Salt and freshly ground pepper to taste
1 large tomato, sliced
10 ounces crumbled non-fat feta cheese
Freshly grated Parmesan cheese (optional)

Heat oil in a large skillet over medium heat; add garlic and onions, sauté until lightly golden. Add eggplant, oregano, and thyme; continue cooking until eggplant browns slightly, stirring constantly. Reduce heat to low, add broth and sherry. Cover and simmer for 3–5 minutes. Stir in salt and pepper to taste if needed, then remove from heat. Allow to cool slightly. Preheat broiler and pour slightly cooled soup into an over-safe bowl. Top soup with tomato slices and feta cheese, place soup under broiler, and heat until feta melts into soup. Garnish with grated Parmesan cheese if desired, and broil again until Parmesan is lightly browned.

Approx. 146 calories per serving

Pizza

Pizza Margherita
(makes an 8-slice, 15-inch pizza)

Thin Crust Pizza Dough

4 Roma tomatoes, thinly sliced

Salt and freshly ground pepper to taste

½ cup yellow sweet pepper, thinly sliced

¾ cup shredded part-skim mozzarella cheese, about 3 ounces

4–5 snipped fresh basil leaves

¼ cup freshly grated Parmesan cheese

1 tablespoon extra-virgin olive oil

Preheat oven to 450 degrees. Follow directions for pizza dough and roll out to a 12–15 inch round. Place dough on a scantly oiled pizza pan. Spread tomatoes on rolled-out dough almost to the edge of the crust. Sprinkle with salt and pepper to taste. Top tomatoes with yellow peppers, mozzarella cheese, basil, Parmesan cheese, and drizzle a scant amount of olive oil over the top. Bake at 450 degrees for 8–10 minutes or until the crust is crisp and cheese is melted.

Approx. 202 calories per slice

Thin Crust Pizza Dough
(makes 8-slices for a 15-inch crust)

1 ⅔ cups unbleached all-purpose flour

½ teaspoon salt

1 package dry active yeast

2 tablespoons extra-virgin olive oil

½ cup warm water

Olive oil to lightly coat pan

Put flour, salt, and yeast in a large bowl and mix with a wooden spoon. Make a well in the center and add oil and water. Gradually work in flour from the sides of the bowl as the mixture becomes smooth, pliable, soft dough.

If too sticky, sprinkle a little more flour into the mixture, but don't make the dough dry. Transfer dough to a lightly floured surface and knead for about 10 minutes; add very small amounts of flour if needed until dough becomes smooth and elastic. Rub a small amount of oil over the surface of the dough, then return it to a clean bowl, cover it with cloth, and place it in a warm area for about 1 hour or until dough doubles in size. Remove dough to a lightly floured surface, knead for an additional 2 minutes, then roll out into a 15-inch round. Place on pizza pan and top with sauce and ingredients of choice. Bake at 425 degrees until crust is crispy.

Approx. 115 calories per slice, crust only

Wraps and Sandwiches

Chickpea Pita Pockets

(makes 8 servings)

1 (15-ounce) can chickpeas, rinsed and drained

1 cup shredded fresh spinach

⅔ cup halved seedless red grapes

½ cup finely chopped red bell pepper

⅓ cup thinly sliced celery

½ medium cucumber, diced

¼ cup finely chopped onion

¼ cup light mayonnaise

1 tablespoon balsamic syrup

½ tablespoon poppy seed

4 (6-inch) whole wheat pita loaf, cut each loaf in half

In a large bowl, combine chickpeas, spinach, grapes, red pepper, celery, cucumber, and onion. Whisk together mayonnaise, balsamic syrup, and poppy seeds. Add poppy seed mixture to chickpea mixture and stir until well blended. Lightly toast pita halves and fill with chickpea filling. Serve.

Approx. 152 calories per serving

Veggie Wrap

(makes 6 servings)

Olive oil cooking spray

2 medium tomatoes, cut into ½-inch thick slices

2 cucumbers, sliced lengthwise into ½-inch thick slices

2 small onions, cut into ½-inch thick slices

1 green bell pepper, cut into strips

2 medium zucchini, sliced lengthwise into ½-inch thick slices

Extra-virgin olive oil to drizzle

¾ tablespoon crumbled dried oregano

¼ tablespoon crumbled dried rosemary

¾ teaspoon dried thyme

½ (7-ounce) can chickpeas, rinsed and drained

¼ teaspoon cumin (optional)

Salt and freshly ground pepper to taste

6 whole wheat flat bread (8–10 inch), warmed

Alfalfa sprouts (optional)

Spray non-stick pan with cooking spray. Place tomatoes, cucumbers, onions, peppers, and zucchini on pan, and drizzle with olive oil. Sprinkle with oregano, rosemary, and thyme, and roast for 15–20 minutes at 425 degrees. Add chickpeas and cumin, plus salt and pepper to taste, and cook an additional 15–20 minutes until tender. Fill warmed flat bread with bean and veggie mix, top with alfalfa sprouts, roll up, and serve.

Approx. 170 per serving

Main Dishes

Linguine and Mixed Seafood

(makes 4–6 servings)

8 ounces natural clam juice

2 cups good dry wine (not cooking wine)

¼ pound baby octopus, cleaned

¼ pound shrimp, peeled and deveined

¼ pound calamari, cleaned, cut into ¼-inch rings

20 mussels, scrubbed and debearded (discard any open mussel)

¼ pound bay scallops

3 tablespoons extra-virgin olive oil

3–4 cloves garlic, minced

¼ teaspoon freshly chopped hot peppers

8 small ripe plum tomatoes, chopped into small chunks

Pinch of low-calorie baking sweetener

½ tablespoon chopped fresh parsley

½ tablespoon chopped fresh oregano

Salt and freshly ground pepper to taste

½ pound linguine

10–12 arugula leaves, chopped

10 pitted Kalamata black olives, halved

In a large deep skillet, add clam juice, wine, octopus, shrimp, calamari, mussels, and scallops. Bring to boil, cover, and reduce heat to simmer, stirring occasionally, until calamari and squid are almost tender. Remove mussels and shell, all but 9–12; set these aside for garnish and return shelled mussels to seafood skillet to keep warm. In a separate skillet, over medium heat, add oil and garlic, and sauté until golden brown. Add hot peppers to garlic mixture, reduce heat to simmer, and cook for 1–2 additional minutes. Add tomatoes, sweetener, parsley, oregano, and salt and pepper to taste, and simmer another 3–4 minutes. Cover to keep warm and set aside. Bring water to a boil, add pasta, and cook pasta until al dente. Remove from heat, drain pasta, and return to pot, drizzling with scant amount of olive oil to keep pasta from sticking together. Set aside. With a slotted spoon, remove seafood from skillet and strain remaining liquid through sieve or cheesecloth. Return seafood and 1 cup of strained liquid to skillet; add pasta and tomato mixture and toss all ingredients. Spoon entire linguini and seafood dish into a large pasta bowl, garnish with chopped arugula, black olives, and remaining unshelled mussels, and serve.

Approx. 375 calories per serving

Grilled Citrus Salmon with Garlic Greens

(makes 4 servings)

¼ cup orange marmalade

2 tablespoons fresh lime juice

2 tablespoons fresh lemon juice

¼ cup low-sodium soy sauce

3 teaspoons grated orange rind

4 (3-ounce) salmon fillets, skin off

2 teaspoons extra-virgin olive oil

2 teaspoons minced garlic

2 (10-ounce) bags of fresh spinach

Scant amount of olive oil to rub fish

Salt and freshly ground pepper to taste

1 teaspoon fresh garlic, mashed to rub on fish

1 heaping tablespoon capers, drained

1 tablespoon balsamic vinegar

4 scallions, white and light green parts, thinly sliced (2–3-inch lengths)

Whisk together marmalade, lime and lemon juices, soy sauce, and orange rind; pour mixture over fillets and marinade for 30 minutes in refrigerator. Prepare grill or preheat broiler. Heat olive oil in a heavy skillet over medium-high heat; add garlic and spinach, one bag at a time, and sauté, stirring often, until spinach is wilted (about 2 minutes). Reduce heat to very low to keep warm. Combine olive oil, salt and pepper, mashed garlic, and capers. Rub mixture into both sides of salmon steaks. Grill the fish or broil 3–4 inches from flame for 2–2 ½ minutes on each side. Set fish aside. Remove spinach from heat and toss with vinegar; divide equally on 4 plates. Add grilled salmon fillet to bed of spinach on each plate and garnish with onions. Serve.

Approx. 250 calories per serving

Chicken Piccata

(makes 4 servings)

2 teaspoons extra-virgin olive oil

4 (3-ounce) skinless, boneless chicken breast fillets, lightly pounded

Salt and freshly ground pepper to taste

3 cloves fresh garlic, minced

1 cup low-sodium, fat-free chicken broth

2 tablespoons dry white wine

4 teaspoons lemon juice

1 tablespoon all-purpose flour

2 tablespoons chopped fresh parsley

1 tablespoon capers

Lemon wedges for garnish

Rinse chicken breast fillets under cold water and pat dry. Place breasts between layers of wax paper and lightly pound fillets with a meat mallet. Lightly sprinkle each fillet with salt and pepper if desired. Heat 1 teaspoon of olive oil in a large heavy-bottomed skillet over medium heat, add chicken fillets, and cook until fillets are lightly browned and centers cooked (juice will run clear). Transfer fillets to a serving platter and put in a low-temperature oven to keep warm. Add remaining teaspoon of oil and garlic to skillet and cook for 30 seconds to soften. Combine chicken broth, wine, lemon juice, and flour in a skillet where chicken was cooked. Stir to blend and continue stirring until mixture thickens. Add parsley and capers to sauce. Remove chicken from oven, place each fillet on a plate, and spoon mixture over fillets. Garnish with lemon wedges. Serve with cooked spinach linguine or pasta of choice.

Approx. 223 calories per serving

Spicy Whole Wheat Capellini with Garlic

(makes 4 servings)

8 ounces whole wheat capellini pasta

¼ cup extra-virgin olive oil

4 cloves garlic, chopped

1 teaspoon diced hot peppers

Salt and freshly ground pepper to taste

Grated Pecorino or Parmesan cheese to taste (optional)

Bring water to boil, add pasta, and cook until al dente. Remove from heat, drain pasta, and return to pot, drizzling with scant olive oil to keep pasta from sticking together. Set aside. In a heavy skillet over medium heat, add olive oil, then sauté garlic and hot pepper until tender (about 1–2 minutes). Add to pasta and toss. Add salt and pepper to taste, and sprinkle with grated cheese if desired.

Approx. 299 calories per serving

Fettuccine with Smoked Salmon and Basil Pesto

(makes 4 servings)

8 ounces dried whole grain fettuccine pasta

Drizzle of extra-virgin olive oil

¼ cup market fresh Basil Pesto Sauce

10 pitted olives, halved

½ tablespoon capers, rinsed well and drained

6 ounces nova smoked salmon (cut into thin strips)

1 tablespoon freshly grated Romano cheese

4 sprigs fresh basil leaves for garnish

Bring water to a boil, add pasta, and cook until al dente. Remove from heat, drain, and return to pot, drizzling with scant amount of olive oil to keep pasta from sticking together. Set aside. Meanwhile, warm pesto sauce in a saucepan under low heat, add olives and capers, remove from heat, and add salmon. In a large serving bowl, toss pasta and salmon mixture. Divide into 4 portions, sprinkle each portion with ¼ tablespoon of Romano cheese, and garnished with fresh basil.

Approx. 323 calories per serving

Fettuccine with Sundried Tomatoes and Goat Cheese

(makes 6-8 servings)

4 tablespoons chopped sundried tomatoes (in olive oil)

1 cup sliced scallions

4 garlic cloves, minced

1 medium red bell pepper, thinly sliced

½ cup dry vermouth

¼ cup chopped fresh basil

10 pitted Kalamata olives

1 tablespoon capers, rinsed and drained

2 teaspoons dried oregano

1 pound whole wheat fettuccine, cooked and drained

6 ounces low-fat goat cheese, crumbled

Drain oil from tomatoes and reserve oil; set tomatoes aside. In a large skillet, heat oil from tomatoes over medium heat. Add scallions and garlic to oil and sauté until soft. Add red peppers and ¼ cup of vermouth to garlic mixture. Cook peppers until crispy tender or until vermouth is almost evaporated. Reduce heat to simmer and add tomatoes, remaining ¼ cup of vermouth, basil, olives, capers, and oregano. Simmer, stirring often to incorporate flavors (about 5–8 minutes), then reduce to very low heat to keep warm. Cook pasta until al dente and drain. Place pasta in a large bowl and toss with goat cheese. Add tomato mixture and toss again until well mixed. Serve.

Approx. 269 calories per serving

Side Dishes

Grilled Eggplant

(makes 4 servings)

1 tablespoon extra-virgin olive oil

2 tablespoons fresh oregano leaves

2 plum tomatoes, diced

1 ½ pounds eggplant, cut lengthwise into ½-inch thick slices

Olive oil cooking spray

2 large garlic cloves, finely minced

1 teaspoon chopped dried rosemary

Salt and freshly ground pepper to taste

¼ crumbled feta cheese

Lemon wedges

Oregano sprigs for garnish

Heat oil in a saucepan, add oregano leaves, then remove pan from heat. Add tomato to oregano and allow to bathe in hot oil until ready to serve. Meanwhile, spray both sides of eggplant with olive oil spray, sprinkle with garlic, rosemary, and salt and pepper, and place on medium-hot grill. Cover grill and cook eggplant until tender and browned on both sides, turning once. Remove eggplant to platter, drizzle with oregano tomato oil, and top with feta cheese. Garnish with lemon wedges and oregano sprigs.

Approx. 74 calories per serving

Roasted Peppers

4 large red bell peppers
2 cloves garlic, peeled and sliced
4 tablespoons extra-virgin olive oil
Salt and freshly ground pepper to taste

Clean peppers and pat dry. Place peppers on moderately hot grill or on a rack under a broiler 1–2 inches from heat, turning often until skin is charred and blistered. Charring of entire skin takes about 15–20 minutes. Remove from grill or broiler and place peppers aside to cool. When cool enough to handle, rub off blackened skins. Cut each pepper in half, remove stalk and seeds, and cut into ½-inch strips. Place strips in a bowl, and add garlic, oil and salt and pepper to taste. Toss and set aside for about 30 minutes before serving.

Approx. 108 calories per serving

Classic Spinach and Pine Nuts

(makes 4 servings)

¼ cup golden raisins

4 tablespoons pine nuts

2 tablespoons extra-virgin olive oil

4 cloves garlic, chopped

1 ½ (10-ounce) bags fresh spinach, cleaned

Salt and freshly ground pepper to taste

Fresh squeezed lemon juice

Place raisins in a bowl and cover with boiling water. Let stand for approximately 10 minutes until raisins are plump; drain well. In a skillet over medium heat, toast pine nuts, stirring constantly for about 1–2 minutes, until toasted. Remove from heat. In a large skillet, warm oil, add garlic and sauté until soft. Add spinach a little at a time, stirring and adding until it is all wilted (about 3–5 minutes). Pour raisins over spinach, add salt and pepper to taste and mix well. With a slotted spoon, transfer spinach to a serving dish, then drizzle with lemon juice and sprinkle with pine nuts. Serve immediately.

Approx. 149 calories per serving

Broccoli with Fresh Garlic

(makes 4–6 servings)

10–12 fresh broccoli spears, roughly 6 inches long

3 cups low-sodium, fat-free chicken broth

3 tablespoons extra-virgin olive oil

2–3 cloves fresh garlic, crushed

2 tablespoons chopped fresh parsley

Salt to taste

Pinch of freshly ground pepper to taste

Cook spears in a large skillet of chicken broth until slightly undercooked (about 7 minutes). Test with a fork; do not overcook. Drain well and set aside. Heat oil in a large skillet over medium-high heat; add garlic and sauté until golden brown. Add broccoli, parsley, and seasonings to taste. Turn broccoli several times, mixing well with seasonings, oil, and garlic. Serve immediately.

Approx. 161 calories per serving

Desserts

Strawberries and Balsamic Syrup

(makes 4 servings)

2 ½ cup strawberries, hulled and halved
4 tablespoons Crème de Banana liqueur
Non-caloric sweetener to taste

Balsamic syrup. Combine strawberries and liqueur in a large bowl, toss well, cover and refrigerate 20–30 minutes. When ready to serve, remove strawberries with a slotted spoon and place in a single layer on a dessert platter. Dust generously with sweetener, drizzle with balsamic syrup, and serve.

Approx. 49 calories per serving

Honeydew Sorbet

(makes 4–6 servings)

1 ½ cups of water

½ cup low-calorie baking sweetener

2 ripe honeydews (about 5 inches in diameter each), peeled, seeded, and chunked

¼ cup fresh lemon juice

¼ cup egg whites

Mint sprigs for garnish

Combine water and sweetener and bring to a boil over medium heat. Reduce heat and simmer for 5 minutes, then allow to cool. In a food processor or blender, add honeydew and its juices, lemon juice, and cooled syrup. Puree until smooth. Pour mixture into bowl and freeze until almost frozen. Remove from freezer and beat with an electric beater until mixture is again smooth. Beat egg white until stiff and fold into frozen fruit mixture. Cover container and freeze again until firm (about 2–3 hours). When ready to serve, scoop into dessert cups and garnish with mint sprigs if desired.

Approx. 117 calories per serving

Meringue Cookies
(makes 20–24 cookies)

1 cup liquid egg whites

Pinch cream of tartar

¼ cup low-calorie baking sweetener

1 teaspoon white wine vinegar

1 teaspoon vanilla extract

Line 2 cookie trays with parchment paper. Place egg whites in a mixing bowl and slowly whisk on low speed with an electric beater until they begin to bubble. Add cream of tartar and increase speed slightly; whisk until the mixture begins to peak. Increase speed to medium and slowly add sweetener, vinegar, and vanilla extract. Continue whisking until mixture is satiny and firmly holds peak. Ladle a soup spoon–sized portion of mixture onto parchment-lined trays to make 20–24 cookies. Put trays of meringues in an over preheated to 275 degrees to bake for 1 hour. Turn off oven and allow cookies to stand in closed oven for an additional hour to dry. When meringues are pierced with a toothpick that comes back dry, they are ready. Transfer cookies to cooling racks to continue to cool.

Approx. 5 calories per cookie

Sweet Plum Compote

(makes 6 servings)

Canola oil cooking spray

3 pounds ripe plums, halved and pitted

¼ cup low-calorie baking sweetener

1 cup water

1 tablespoon Crème de Cassis liqueur

Lightly spray a baking dish with cooking spray. Add plums to baking dish. Combine sweetener and water in a saucepan and bring to a boil; cook for about 5 minutes, stirring constantly, or until liquid becomes syrupy. Pour syrup over plums and drizzle with Crème de Cassis. Bake mixture for 45 minutes to 1 hour in a 350-degree oven. Serve warm or cool.

Approx. 130 calories per serving

Peach Marsala Compote
(makes 6 servings)

Canola oil cooking spray

12 fresh peaches

6 cups water

¾ cup low-calorie baking sweetener

½ Marsala wine

½ teaspoon ground cinnamon

½ teaspoon vanilla extract

½ teaspoon freshly grated nutmeg

Lightly spray a 2-quart baking dish with cooking spray. Blanch the peaches in boiling water for 20 seconds, then remove the skin while holding under cold running water. Pit and slice peaches. Add peaches, sweetener, wine, cinnamon, vanilla extract, and nutmeg to a baking dish and bake for 45 minutes to 1 hour in a 350-degree over. Serve warm or at room temperature.

Approx. 80 calories per serving

Strawberries Amaretto

(makes 8 servings)

3 pints fresh strawberries

2 cups plain low-fat yogurt

1 teaspoon vanilla extract

¼ cup Amaretto liqueur

Fat-free whipped cream (if desired)

Set aside 8 strawberries for garnish. Hull remaining strawberries and cut into halves. Place strawberry halves in dessert cups. In a bowl combine yogurt, vanilla extract, and liqueur; blend well. Pour over strawberries and garnish each cup with a reserved berry. Add whipped cream if desired.

Approx. 96 calories per serving

Fresh Fruit Kabobs and Cinnamon Honey Dip

(makes 2 servings)

Assorted bite-sized chunks of your favorite fresh fruits (enough for 2 [8-inch] wooden skewers)

1 cup of plain low-fat Greek yogurt

2 tablespoons of honey or non-caloric sweetener

Pinch of ground white pepper

6 teaspoons of ground cinnamon or to taste

Prepare fruits on skewers and set aside. Combine yogurt, honey, and white pepper, and mix well. Divide mixture into two individual serving bowls; sprinkle cinnamon on top of each serving and gently swirl in. Cover and refrigerate to chill before serving.

NOTE: Values shown are for yogurt dip only (values for fruit cannot be calculated since they depend on the specific fruits chosen).

Approx. 70 calories per serving

Restaurant Survival Guide

Certainly cooking recipes at home is the best way to know what you are eating is good for you, both body-friendly and heart-healthy. So what do you do when you go out to a restaurant or head to your friend's house for a dinner party? Worse, what happens at the holidays?

Don't fear. You can take the Mediterranean diet and all of its health benefits on the road with you and still have a wonderful time. And who knows, maybe you will leave a healthful impression on your friends.

Just use these easy-to-follow recommendations:

- Don't go to a restaurant when you are starving. Drink a glass of water and enjoy a handful of almonds before you go. That way, you won't be tempted to devour the breadbasket while you're waiting for your meal.
- Speaking of that breadbasket, ask for whole grain bread and olive oil if white bread and butter arrives. But remember, if you're watching your calories, a tablespoon of olive oil has 120 calories,

so use it sparingly and mix with a little balsamic vinegar for flavor.

- Load up on vegetables. Don't be afraid to order a healthy mixed vegetable salad as an appetizer. But always order the dressing on the side, or better yet, just ask for olive oil and vinegar on the table. That way you can control the amount, and you know it is the healthiest option. Believe me, you won't miss that heavy ranch or processed Thousand Island.
- For a protein or main dish, opt for skinless poultry or fish over red meat.
- And choose foods that are baked, broiled, or grilled; nothing fried.
- Steer clear of processed foods. Fresh food is always healthier, and it tastes much better too!
- Be certain your foods are not being cooked with the preservative MSG or trans fats (hydrogenated oils). Do not be afraid to ask to be sure!
- When ordering pasta or pizzas, ask for whole grain versions. Most restaurants will have it.
- Choose brown rice over white rice.
- Avoid fruit drinks and sodas. Unsweetened iced tea, especially green tea, is always a good option if you want a change from water.
- Always leave a little on the plate. You're an adult! No one will ever make you clean your plate again, so see how full you are after eating

half of your portion. If you feel full, then take the other half home.

- Alternatively, ask for half of your portion to be wrapped up ahead of time!
- Order fresh fruit for dessert, or the dessert that has fresh fruit with it.
- Consider hot herbal tea after your meal.

About the Author

Michael Ozner, MD, FACC, FAHA, is one of America's leading advocates for heart disease prevention. Ozner is a board-certified cardiologist, a Fellow of both the American College of Cardiology and the American Heart Association, Medical Director of Wellness and Prevention at Baptist 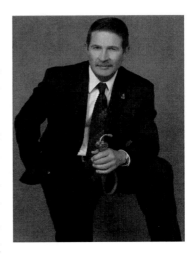 Health South Florida, and a well-known regional and national speaker in the field of preventive cardiology. He is symposium director for "Cardiovascular Disease Prevention," an annual international meeting dedicated to the treatment and prevention of heart attack and stroke. Dr. Ozner was the past president of the American Heart Association of Miami and the recipient of the American Heart Association Humanitarian Award. He was elected to "Top Cardiologists in America" by the Consumer Council of America. Dr. Ozner is also the author of *The Great American Heart Hoax, Heart Attack Proof,* and *The Complete Mediterranean Diet.*

To contact Dr. Ozner, visit www.DrOzner.com.